Prepare yourself for the powerful storytelling of Sophie Jackson . . .

Sophie Jackson is an English teacher from Chorley. Although she read and wrote furiously as a child, she first started writing as an adult, to scratch the creative itch, for the website FanFiction.net, after reading the *Twilight* series in 2008. She wrote and posted a number of *Twilight* fanfics, chapter by chapter, and built up an impressive readership.

For more information, visit Sophie's website www.sophiejacksonauthor.com and find her on Facebook at www.facebook.com/SophieJacksonRomance and on Twitter @sophiejax.

Praise for Sophie Jackson's intoxicating romances:

'Entirely heartfelt, hot and should be the very next book on your TBR list' *Romantic Times*

'[Sophie] writes the type of stories today's reader wants: beautifully created characters filled with emotion, and a storyline that sticks with you long after you turn the last page' *Tara Sue Me*

'This book truly was outstanding and I can't express just how much I loved reading it. It's the kind of book that I felt in my chest and made me angry when life got in the way of my reading' *Holly's Red Hot Reviews*

'Sophie weaves storylines to build suspense before everything ultimately comes together, leaving the reader guessing and gasping until the very end' *J. M. Darhower*

By *Sophie Jackson*

A Pound of Flesh Series
A Pound of Flesh
Love and Always (e-novella)
An Ounce of Hope

an ounce of
hope

SOPHIE JACKSON

headline
ETERNAL

The right of Sophie Jackson to be identified as the Author of
the Work has been asserted by her in accordance with the
Copyright, Designs and Patents Act 1988.

Published by arrangement with Gallery Books,
a division of Simon & Schuster, Inc.

First published in Great Britain in 2016
by HEADLINE ETERNAL
An imprint of HEADLINE PUBLISHING GROUP

1

All characters in this publication are fictitious
and any resemblance to real persons, living or dead,
is purely coincidental.

Cataloguing in Publication Data is available from the British Library

ISBN 978 1 4722 2466 8

Offset in 10.75/15 pt Adode Garamond Pro by Jouve (UK)

Printed and bound by CPI Group (UK) Ltd, Croydon, CR0 4YY

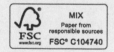

Headline's policy is to use papers that are natural, renewable and recyclable
products and made from wood grown in well-managed forests and other
controlled sources. The logging and manufacturing processes are expected
to conform to the environmental regulations of the country of origin.

HEADLINE PUBLISHING GROUP
An Hachette UK Company
Carmelite House
50 Victoria Embankment
London EC4Y 0DZ

www.headlineeternal.com
www.headline.co.uk
www.hachette.co.uk

For the most amazing fandom, my online family.
You are all of you amazing. Don't ever change.

ACKNOWLEDGMENTS

As always, special thanks to my incredible team—a group of women who inspire me and keep me sane every day: Lorella and Louise, who are the most awesome pair of agents; Micki, Marla, and Kristin at Gallery Books; and Kate and Jo at Headline Eternal. My gratitude for all you do is immeasurable.

To my family, my friends, and to everyone else who has read, reviewed, retweeted, liked, blogged, and recommended these books. Your enthusiasm and love for these characters makes writing them an absolute joy.

You are the milk to my Oreo, and I adore each and every one of you.

Hope is like the sun, which, as we journey toward it, casts the shadow of our burden behind us.

—Samuel Smiles

1

The first time Max O'Hare thought about taking his life was the day of his father's funeral. It was a bleak mid-October morning, the kind where wind whips at your face, and rain doesn't fall, but pours in torrents and makes even the most happy-go-lucky of assholes consider what the hell they were cheerful about in the first place.

Max had watched them lower his father's casket into the ground, right next to Hazel O'Hare's, Max's mother. The beautiful headstone above her plot, which showed in stunning gold lettering how she was only twenty-six when she was killed in a head-on collision on her way to her son's second birthday party, now had a neighbor. After a courageous eighteen-month battle with pancreatic cancer, Connor O'Hare had finally succumbed to the cruel disease at the age of forty-five, leaving Max an orphan.

An orphan who couldn't help but wonder just what the fuck he was meant to do with his life.

Sure, there was the family business, a specialist auto body shop where Max had learned his father's trade as a mechanic with an enthusiastic eye and a hero-worshipping ear, but that shit became superfluous when Connor was no longer able to work. The fuck hot muscle cars and the roaring engines; none of it mattered. All that mattered was when the next round of chemo was, and what ridiculous figure the medical bills were amounting to.

Not that Max's father ever complained or worried about that. He'd smile when Max started to stress about appointments and money, and tell him life was too damned short to sweat the small stuff. But that was the way Connor O'Hare was. Maybe that's why he never lost his shit when, as a teenager, Max was brought home numerous times in a police cruiser, or when he was arrested for dope possession and car boosting. You'll find your way, his father would say with a disappointed shrug that made Max's teeth grind in guilt; these are just bumps in the road, son.

Max wasn't so sure, but similarly, he didn't know why he got into the shit he did. Boredom maybe? Hell, he couldn't even use having a shitty home life as an excuse. His father was a good man who did his best raising his son alone. No. Max was a law unto himself, his own worst enemy. He wished to be strong like his dad, noble and dedicated, but he failed every damned time.

True to form, Max's father's battle against his illness was valiant, and he stayed brave to the very end, but his death wasn't that of a warrior. It wasn't romantic. There were no whispered words of love or declarations of life lessons and regret, what with him being unable to speak—the cancer had affected his lungs and throat by then. Max simply watched his father become more and more ravaged by an illness, which stole away the tough vibrancy he'd known and respected. All that was left was an aged shell of a man who slipped away in his sleep while Max held his hand from his permanent vigil at the side of the hospital bed.

Such was the grief that gripped Max, that he didn't even cry. His eyes stayed resolutely dry, as though sorrow blocked every part of him, every tear duct, vein, and artery. Yeah, that shit was grim.

He had friends around him, of course. Friends—who were more like family—and were prepared to bend over backward for him. *Anything we can do. I'm here if you want to talk.* Jesus, he could barely get out of bed in the morning and they were expecting him to talk. He appreciated it, sure, but their words were breaths on a breeze that, as time passed, continued to guide Max into a dark depression. That darkness culminated in his downing a bottle of vodka and snorting a dozen lines of coke, while staring passively at a bottle of pills he'd found among his father's things.

It'd be so easy, he'd thought.

So fucking easy.

And painless.

That's what he wanted above all other things: a pain-free existence.

But he hadn't gone through with it. Cowardice was not something Max was proud of, but, like his best friend, Carter, had explained: he was twenty years old and had his whole life to live. And live it he did. He got shitfaced, fucked women, dealt in shit he had no business getting involved in, became a regular dealer, got shot at, got arrested, got bailed . . . rinse and repeat.

Not a life so much as an extended hangover, punctuated with pockets of deliriousness. He kept the body shop afloat with the money he made from dealing, paid his employees, and partied from sunset to sunrise. And as the months passed, the pain Max had felt the day of the funeral slowly ebbed, leaving a numbness in which he freely basked. He didn't feel pain. Christ, he didn't feel anything. And that was just fine.

He doubted he'd ever feel again. He wasn't sure he even wanted to.

Until *she* tumbled into his life . . .

Max lifted his eyes from the sumptuous cream carpet under his feet, settling them on the man sitting opposite him. Elliot waited patiently for Max to say something else, but Max knew he was done. He'd said more than he'd wanted to already. He hadn't spoken about his father for a long time and scratching at that particular scab was as agonizing as it had been on the day of the funeral eight years before.

He reached for the glass of water on the small wooden table at the side of his chair and took a long sip. The silence was suffocating in its expectancy, causing Max to fidget and shift in his seat.

"From your quiet, I assume we're done for the day." Elliot smiled and wrote quickly on the legal pad resting, as it always did, on his knee. Max didn't answer, but took a deep breath, knowing he'd been let off the hook. Max had learned quickly that Dr. Elliot Watts was a persistent bastard. Yeah, he was a therapist and that shit was his job, but he'd been relentless from the get-go. Nevertheless, Max had to admit he liked him, no matter what dark paths of the past the doc asked him to travel.

"You made some good progress here today, Max," Elliot continued with a small nod. "I know talking about your father isn't easy."

Yeah, no shit.

Scribble, scribble. "So, you're fifteen days in. How are you finding the medication?"

Max shrugged. He was on a plethora of funky-looking pills, which he had to take each morning: antidepressants, Ritalin, amantadine. Each one had a very specific purpose in helping with the aching despair, sleepless nights, and the cravings. And they did. For the most part. Hell, drugs were drugs.

They weren't the drugs he wanted, the drugs he knew would kick his anxiety's ass, the drugs that would stop his dick from being a flaccid waste of time, the drugs that would supress the monstrous appetite that was adding to his waistline, the drugs that beckoned like a fucking siren's call every time he tried to close his eyes at night.

But drugs were drugs.

With every half-assed beat of his heart, his blood moved sluggishly around his body. It was desperate for the fire of a line, the life, the euphoric detachment. Jesus, he needed a hit. Just one fucking hit.

Elliot sat up a little straighter, as if sensing the hunger that practically crippled Max from the inside out. "How are the night terrors?"

Dread seized Max's bones. He swallowed and rubbed his hands

together. His discomfort spoke volumes. The night terrors were just that: terrifying. Nightmares so vivid and distressing the mere thought of sleep left Max cold. They'd started just days off the powder, just days after he'd been admitted, and, despite Elliot's prescribed medication, they weren't abating. The bags under his eyes could attest to that shit.

"We can increase the dose if you need it, Max," Elliot said softly. "You need your rest."

Max sighed and gave an imperceptible dip of his chin, his pride unable to outweigh the fear of what waited for him when he slept.

"Okay. I'll get that changed for you."

"Thank you." Max's voice was quiet, but his gratitude was immeasurable.

"Do you want to talk about the terrors?"

"No." Max rubbed at his temples, where the grotesque images that accosted him at night threatened to claw out.

Elliot's silence made Max lift his head. "That bad."

Max pulled the hood of his sweatshirt farther around his face, burying himself in an attempt to hide. He wore his hood up for both his individual and the group sessions, and weirdly, Elliot didn't seem to mind. Max wasn't entirely sure why he did it, but it helped take the edge off the stress he felt at the thought of talking to strangers about shit that had happened years ago. It was a cocoon, a wall that made his stay in rehab a little bit easier.

"Maybe you could write about the terrors in the notebook I gave you last week. I know it's still empty." Elliot smiled wryly at the derisive look Max shot him.

Writing in a fucking notebook? No, thanks.

"Fine, look," Elliot said, sitting forward, "you know where I am if you want to talk more. We're all here to help you through this. You're not alone, okay?"

Max scoffed inwardly, holding his eye roll. Sure, he was surrounded by people who had his "very best interests at heart," people who wanted to "help him get clean," wanted to "talk it all out together," wanted to make sure that he was "comfortable," "at ease," and not frantic with the need to bust out of the fucking place and find the nearest junkie stash.

Yeah, he was well and truly surrounded by well-meaning folk. And he'd never felt more alone.

2

Seven years ago . . .

The party, as they always did, had descended into chaos. It was nearly midnight and Riley Moore, flanked by three of his friends, was—using only his teeth to lift the glasses—shooting vodka shots off the naked breasts of two unnamed girls. Max smiled as the guys cheered and whooped, high-fived and chest-bumped with each shot that spilled gloriously over the skin of the girls, chased by Riley's eager tongue.

Max laughed at the enthusiastic cleanup job. Meeting through mutual friends, Max had only known Riley for a couple of years. Nevertheless, Max had learned pretty quickly that, despite not knowing too much about the man's background, Riley was always the life and soul of any shindig and was a monster when it came to drinking. He drank damned near anything as long as it was alcoholic, yet always seemed to stay resolutely sober no matter how many bottles sat around him. He was crazy, but he never touched anything else. Not even weed. Riley always turned it down, saying it never interested him. Max had always been silently in awe of his self-restraint.

No, Riley's vices were cars and women. Lots of women.

Max's elbow was bumped hard. He turned to see his best friend, Carter, high and drunk, with his arm wrapped around a cute brunette who was wearing very little.

"Cheer up, man," Carter said with a wide smile. "Come on. It's a party."

Max nodded and lifted his beer bottle, tipping the neck toward his friend. "I'm all good," he replied, draining his beer, knowing that the line he'd done not an hour before was losing its edge. "Can you hit me up?"

Carter nodded and fumbled in his jeans pocket, pulling out a small Baggie. "Have at it, my friend, and then get drunk, get laid, get something to put a smile on your fucking face!"

Max laughed as he watched Carter stumble over to one of the couches, where he collapsed with his new friend and began sucking face. Bastard was right, though. Max was almost twenty-two years old. He needed to cut loose, have some real fun, and snap out of the grief that still hung around his neck after the loss of his father a year and a half before. He just didn't know how to do it without a couple of lines and a beer. He knew his partying was teetering on the very edge of dangerous, but, ironically enough, that thrill alone kept Max's nose in the powder and a drink in his hand.

"You came!" The squealing sound of one of the half-naked vodka shots girls brought Max's head up from the bag in his hand. The skinny redhead scrambled from the table, pulling on her T-shirt—much to the annoyance of the men in the immediate vicinity—and hurried across the apartment to the open doorway.

Max watched her with a small smile that immediately dropped when he saw the girl she was greeting. Jesus. She was . . . tall and blonde. Very blonde. And natural blonde, too. That shit wasn't out of a bottle. It was honey and ash and sat on petite shoulders dressed in a red short-sleeved top. The jeans she wore were black and clung to her legs like a second skin. She was . . . Christ, she was lovely.

"Come and meet Riley! We've been doing naked shots!" Redhead bounced on the balls of her feet, dragging the intriguing new addition back toward the kitchen.

From Blonde's expression, as she looked around the mayhem, Max could tell she wasn't the type of girl who would disrobe and allow random men to shoot drinks off her tits. Bizarrely, that thought comforted an unfamiliar spot in Max's chest. She was lithe and elegant as she crossed the room, and Max found himself craning his neck to watch her over and around the other people at the party. People he'd forgotten about, didn't give a shit about.

"Riley, this is my best friend, Lizzie. Lizzie, meet Riley." Redhead draped herself over Riley's arm while Lizzie smiled.

And what a fucking smile it was.

All white teeth, sparkle, and fucking rainbows.

"Hey, Liz." Riley grinned. "You want a drink?"

"It's Lizzie, and, no, I don't drink and drive," she remarked. Max chuckled at her sass and the surprised look on Riley's face.

Riley's laughter exploded out of him. "Well, shit, Lizzie, let me get you a Sprite at the very least."

Before she could respond, Riley had poured her a Sprite and handed it to her with a wink. The smirk that graced Lizzie's face was sexy as hell. Max shifted closer to where they all stood, pushing the forgotten bag of coke into his back pocket, his attention well and truly diverted.

He observed Lizzie for the forty minutes she stayed, captivated. She was charming and funny, giving as good as she got when the banter started in earnest. She even glanced in Max's direction a few times. He smiled gently and nodded in reaction. The pink hue that lit her cheeks when he did was delicious.

Ordinarily, Max would have been at her side chatting up a storm with charismatic lines of flowery shit that, experience had taught him, chicks loved.

But something held him back. Something foreign and scary. Something that told him this Lizzie would hand him his balls if he tried to be anything but real and honest.

So he watched, knowing as she left that he had to see her again.

. . .

The grounds of the rehab center were vast. Fifteen acres, to be exact. Before the south-central Pennsylvania snow had gotten too deep, Max had meandered about the lands, stopped for a smoke, and meandered some more. The quiet was ear piercing and made him twitchy as all get-out. He was used to the hustle and bustle of New York City life, and the sprawling fields and fresh air were hard to get used to.

When he wasn't at one of his fifteen sessions a week with Elliot, with his sobriety counselor, or wandering aimlessly, Max sat in his room, listened to music, or read. And that was just fine when he was going through the initial cocaine withdrawals, which were fucking *awesome* and slowed him down to a damned snail's pace. Two weeks on, however, and he was starting to get itchy feet. Elliot had promised that, once he'd plateaued on his meds, Max could start working out with a personal trainer. Frankly, Max was dying to get into the gym to work off some of the tension and stress that curled his shoulders inward. But he had to wait. As an alternative, Max was offered the chance to join a yoga class.

Something slow. Something easy.

He'd laughed in Elliot's face. No, he'd explained. He wasn't a yoga type of guy. Instead, he'd retired back to his room.

Not that he minded being in his room. And honestly, "room" was a broad term. It was more like a hotel suite. It was fixed up sweet with a huge bed, comfortable chairs, nice artwork on the walls, and an en suite bathroom. Apparently Carter had picked the joint because of its more relaxed, homey vibe, as well as it being small with only seventeen "clients" at any one time, ensuring one-on-one, twenty-four-hour care and support. Max knew Carter had paid through the nose to get him in on such short notice.

Although the Narcotics Anonymous twelve steps to recovery were very much part of Max's healing process, the facility also offered more holistic-type therapy, which Max was sure would benefit someone. Just not him. He wasn't into all that mind, body, and soul mumbo jumbo. He just wanted to get clean the fastest way possible so he could go home.

Still, after fifteen days, Max had to admit, somewhat begrudgingly, that rehab wasn't all bad. He missed his friends and the comforts of home like crazy, of course, but it was kind of like being in prison. Only cozier. With nicer smells, nicer drapes, and easier smiles from the staff. Sure, the sessions with Elliot were a heinous chore that made Max want to do nothing but go fetal, and the group sessions were even worse, but the guys he'd met in group had definitely made his stay more interesting. Talk about crackpots.

Take Stan, for example. Stan was twenty-eight years old and a coke addict. Like Max, he'd delved into the white powder time and time again as a way of forgetting life and all the bullshit that came with it. He was a five-foot-six, tenacious Puerto Rican who could talk the hind legs off a motherfucking donkey. And he did. Regularly. But that was just fine with Max. If Stan was talking, that meant Lyle, the group leader, and Hud, a sobriety counselor, weren't looking in Max's direction expecting *him* to say anything.

For the ten group sessions the seventeen of them had had, Max still hadn't spoken a word. Didn't *want* to speak a word. Didn't know where the hell he'd start putting that shit in organized, fluent sentences. Jesus, being sober and lucid did nothing but encourage his once-quieted thoughts to relentlessly hammer his tortured brain from the minute he opened his eyes every morning. The luscious coke blanket he'd used unashamedly every day, numerous times a day, to silence the fuckery taking place in his head was a distant memory. Max simply pulled the substitute blanket—the hood of his sweater—farther around his face, burrowing deeper into the fabric, and tried to relax.

Easier said than done with Stan waxing lyrical about his regrets. Oh, the regrets.

"I swear to fucking God, does he never shut up?"

Max's eyes slid across to the owner of the whispered complaint, Dom Hayes, another fellow cokehead with a history of dealing, misdemeanors, time inside for stupid shit, etc. He was twenty-six and, his criminal history notwithstanding, a fairly stand-up guy. He'd shared his smokes with Max on one of the first days at the joint when Max was about ready to bust out of the place and beat a hasty retreat back across the state of Pennsylvania, home. They'd been tight ever since. Interestingly enough, Dom reminded Max a lot of Carter, which was as unbearable as it was comforting.

Christ, Max missed his best friend.

Even if Carter was an asshole. An asshole who had been there for Max for nearly twenty years. An asshole who had done time in Arthur Kill prison for Max when shit went tits up. An asshole Max had pulled a gun on when he'd finally hit rock bottom. An asshole who, at the end of his patience, had picked an unconscious Max up off the bathroom floor and begged and yelled at him to get a grip, to go to rehab and get clean. An asshole who drove him for nearly four hours to the rehab facility, paid for everything without question, and hugged him hard before he left with tears in his eyes, telling Max that everything would be all right.

Max sighed and closed his eyes briefly, zoning out Stan and the other seventeen men in the room. Max knew that, without Carter, he'd be dead. He knew that, without Carter's finances and Riley's business know-how, his father's auto shop would have been lost along with the reputation his dad had worked so damned hard to build. Without Carter, Max would never have survived losing Lizzie.

As always happened when he thought about her, severe pain sliced through Max's stomach, up to his chest, clutching his heart and lungs, causing him to sit forward in his seat. He gasped through the unrelenting agony, thankful that everyone's attention was still on Stan.

Everyone's except Dom's. "You okay, man?" he muttered at his side.

Max nodded, cleared his throat, and tried to breathe just the way Elliot had shown him. Slow and steady. Deep and gradual. In. Out. In. Out.

Once such a simple motion and now, without her, and without any white lines, an enduring struggle.

. . .

"So tell me about your episode in group."

Max was starting to realize that Dr.. Elliot was fucking omniscient or some shit. Nothing got past him. Bastard must have cameras in every part of the damned center. He knew everything! Either that or his small "episode" in group wasn't as subtle as Max had hoped.

He shrugged. "It was nothing."

Why he continued to lie, God alone knew. It certainly didn't make him feel any better and it certainly wasn't going to get his ass home any sooner. And wasn't that the endgame, to get better and then get home?

Scribble. Scribble. "Max, it will help to talk about it." Elliot sipped from his always-present Phillies mug. Max wondered if it was coffee or something stronger, like cognac. Or whiskey. Dammit, a shot of Jack would have been a real fucking treat right about then.

"It was the same as before," Max murmured with a slow exhale.

Elliot's eyes softened. "Lizzie."

Max's chest gave an ungrateful squeeze at the sound of the two syllables.

"Tell me," Elliot said quietly. "Whatever you can. Tell me."

Whether it was the soft coaxing of Elliot's voice, or the need to show everyone he could recover, or whether it was the urgent need Max had to not let Carter down, the cracks in his emotional dam slowly started to give way. He began by telling Elliot about the party, the first time he'd seen *her* and not spoken to her because he'd been too chickenshit. The lighthearted abuse he'd received from Riley and Carter because he wouldn't pick up the phone and call her for weeks after, despite his desperate need to see her again. Jesus, the need. The need that still crippled him. Fuck, and then there was the sound of her soft, eager voice when he'd finally plucked up the courage to dial the digits written on the battered piece of paper he'd had in his pocket since Riley's shindig. Their first date at a bowling alley where she whipped his ass by nearly fifty points and then let him kiss her. The kiss, her lips . . .

. . . Max could barely breathe. His chest constricted as the memories pummeled him in torrents, unyielding and fierce. His heart thundered in his chest, causing his vision to tunnel and his face to burn. He had to get out of that fucking office, but his brain couldn't send the signals to his feet quick enough. And there was pain in his chest. He rubbed at it, while trying to tell Elliot that he thought there was a high chance he was having a heart attack. But no words came from his breathless mouth.

He didn't see Elliot move, but there he was, kneeling at Max's side, imploring him to breathe deeply, calmly gripping his fore-arm. Although Max could feel his psychiatrist's urgent fingers, he couldn't answer. The panic choked him. It was almost funny. Here was his shrink, begging for Max to talk, to open up, and the one time Max wanted to, he couldn't. Now, that shit was ironic. He collapsed in his chair, aware of voices, but unable to respond. It was almost as though he was outside of himself; floating above his body, watching the tsunami of emotion drown him.

And that was his last thought before the jaws of suffocation consumed him completely: I'm dying.

3

"I was wondering when you'd call."

Max blinked. "You were? But . . . how did you know I got your number?"

She laughed. It was a lush, sweet sound that made Max smile. "Riley may have told Amber. Amber told me."

"Amber?" Max frowned. "Oh, you mean body shots girl."

She laughed again. "That would be her."

Max chuckled. "Fuckin' Riley."

The silence that overtook the phone line was hesitant but exciting. Max's mouth was suddenly very dry. He pinched the bridge of his nose, silently pleading for a rush of testosterone or something to help him grow some balls and ask the girl out.

"So you called . . ." Lizzie prompted.

"Yes!" Max exclaimed quickly. "Yes, I did. I . . . well, I didn't get a chance to speak to you at the party the other week and—"

"Yeah, you stood on the other side of the room smiling at me all night and never made a move. Were you waiting for an invitation?"

Max barked a laugh. Her attitude was incredibly sexy. "Well, damn, woman, don't go easy on me, huh?"

Her laugh got louder. "I won't! Am I really that scary?"

"No! No, you're gorgeous, I mean, you know, and not scary and, fuck, I mean, I just, well, you were with your friends and I didn't want to interrupt."

"Max?"

The way she said his name made the muscles in his stomach tighten. "Yeah?"

"I'd love to go on a date with you."

•   •   •

Max awoke slowly. Sounds, smells, and sensations nudged him into consciousness, where, for two awesome seconds, he forgot that he was a zillion miles from home and in a strange bed. Wait. He was in bed? He glanced around. Yep, he was back in his room. What the hell? The last he remembered, he was in Elliot's office—

"You had a panic attack."

Max startled at the sound of Elliot's voice. He lifted his head from the sumptuous pillow and, through tired eyes, searched the room for him. Elliot was sitting in one of the fancy, high-backed chairs on the far side of the room, right leg crossed over left, watching him carefully.

"I gave you a shot of midazolam, which made you sleep." He waved a hand, gesturing to the bed. "I thought you'd be more comfortable in here, rather than the sofa in my office."

Max rubbed his face, a dull ache tapping at his forehead. "Great." He sat up gradually, his surroundings swimming. "I forgot how fun they could be."

Elliot didn't miss a beat. "You've had panic attacks before?"

Not like that.

Elliot nodded into the ensuing silence, his jaw twitching. "It can be caused by any number of things. In your case I think a combination of your low blood sugar and the topic of conversation contributed to an attack of considerable severity." He sat forward. "You need to make sure your hypoglycemia is under control, Max."

"I know." Max's appetite had been through the damned roof thanks to his coke withdrawals and his meds and, despite the clucking of the kitchen staff, he'd been eating all the wrong shit and not testing his bloods regularly. He just ate. And ate. Dammit, he'd be going back to New York looking like the fucking Pillsbury Doughboy. *Hoo-hoo!*

"Check bloods. Eat better," he muttered. "Got it. Anything else?"

"Yes," Elliot replied sharply. He stood quickly from his seat and approached the bed.

Unused to hearing Elliot so annoyed, and feeling less than golden, Max snapped, "What's your problem, Doc?" Elliot was usually so calm, so passive.

"I don't have a problem, Max," he replied quietly. "You do."

Max snorted. "I only have one? You need to get with the program, man."

Elliot ignored his attempts at levity. He crossed his arms over his chest and looked at Max in a way that made him want to hide under the covers of his bed. "Do you realize that today was the first time since you were admitted that you spoke at length about your past, about Lizzie?"

Max swallowed the bile that crept up his throat.

"Max, brief comments about your father aside, today you unleashed a decade of grief in fifteen minutes. Grief that's been sitting inside of you, festering, buried under a quick wit, a ton of coke, and emotionless fucking."

Despite the truth in Elliot's words, Max blanched. "Jeez, Doc, say it how it is, why dontcha?"

"Like a broken levee, your emotions came out too quickly for your mind to cope. It overwhelmed you and your body panicked. Max, you were barely coherent." Elliot exhaled, never taking his stern stare from his patient. "You can't continue to do this, Max. You *must* start opening up, talking, expressing yourself in *some* way."

Max huffed and dropped his head back against the wall, wishing he could have another shot of whatever funky juice Elliot had given him, just so he could lose himself once more to oblivion.

He'd rather that, he'd rather anything than having to talk about . . . well, everything.

"What if I'm not built that way?" Max was surprised at how quiet his voice was, as he asked the question that had been plaguing him since his first therapy session. He looked up at Elliot. "What if I can't?"

Elliot shook his head slowly. "You can. Together we can. I'll help you every step of the way, Max, we all will, but you have to start meeting us halfway. Lyle is concerned about your insistence to pass on speaking in group—"

"And what if I just don't want to, huh, Doc? What if I just don't want to fucking speak to any of you?"

Elliot stayed silent for an immeasurable amount of time, causing Max to twitch. "But you do want to, Max," he murmured finally. "You're here. You're here because you want to get better. You haven't left because Carter would be devastated and you don't want to disappoint anyone, least of all him. You're here because deep down you know that this is your last chance, your last hope to be clean, happy, and free of all that weighs you down every damn day."

Well, shit. Max's chin hit his chest and a long, slow breath shuddered from him. He rubbed his face, hiding the tears that suddenly welled in his eyes. "Don't pretend like you know me," he muttered, making Elliot chuckle and sigh.

"Tomorrow you have an appointment with Tate Moore."

Max lifted his head, the name ringing some far-off bell of familiarity. "Tate Moore?"

Elliot nodded. "He's one of our part-time resident physicians; he's excellent. He also runs the art classes three days a week."

Max rolled his eyes. "Art classes."

Great. So Elliot was handing him over to some Renoir-loving asshat who no doubt balked at the mere mention of the word "abstract." Not that he had anything against Renoir, but still.

"If you don't like it, you can try something else," Elliot said, all but reading Max's thoughts. "But I want you to engage, express yourself, and communicate. Besides, I remember reading on your admittance form that you liked painting."

Max shrugged. "Carter wrote that. I haven't done it for a long time. I used to paint the cars that came into the shop when I was younger. Then I took my work onto the buildings of New York. Dad used to brag about how his kid could paint the entire island of Manhattan single-handedly . . ." His words caught in his throat.

Elliot placed a hand on his shoulder and squeezed gently. "Paint what you can't say, Max."

Max cocked an eyebrow, dismissing the kind gesture. "And if I don't?"

Elliot stood up straight. "Then I withhold your gym pass." He turned on his heel, leaving Max gaping at the back of him.

"But . . . you said that— Hold the fuck on, Doc!"

"Two weeks," Elliot said calmly from the door. "Two weeks with Tate, improvement in group, and I'll allow you to start working out with a trainer. Deal?"

Max slumped against the pillows. He may have pouted like a child, but he knew he had little choice. "Deal."

. . .

The art room was nothing like Max expected. It was huge, light, airy, and reeked of paint and soap, punctuated by the underlying but instantly recognizable aroma of paint stripper. It was a heady smell that knocked Max headlong into a nostalgic memory of working in his father's shop, spraying the Mustangs and Buicks while rock music shook the entire building. His father loved rocking out to Pink Floyd and the Who. The louder the better, he'd say—

"And you must be Max."

Max turned. The man in the doorway, although older than

Max, was young. Younger than he'd anticipated. He was tall and broad, had dark blond hair that was trimmed closely to his head, large hazel eyes, and an even bigger smile. He held out his left hand, while his right gripped the top of a dark wood cane.

"I'm Tate Moore." They shook hands. "Elliot set up our meeting today." He noticed Max's gaze on the cane. "Eh, the chicks dig a guy with a cane and a limp, what can I say?"

Max pushed his hands into his pockets, his eyes wary. "You're the art guy?"

Tate grinned. "Not what you were expecting, huh?"

The guy was wearing black jeans, Converse, and a T-shirt that, underneath the outline of a Tardis, read "Trust Me I'm The Doctor."

Max shook his head. "Not really."

Tate waved a hand dismissively. "I get that a lot." He walked into the room, past Max. In fairness, the man's limp wasn't so bad. "We have the place to ourselves for a little while before my next sitting. Tell me about art."

Max frowned. "Huh?"

Tate smiled as he settled onto a rolling stool, propping his cane against his thigh. "What's your experience? Are you a beginner? What do you favor? Paints, pencils, charcoal? Tell me."

Max glanced out the large French windows, which looked out onto the snow-covered land of the center. "I like paints. I painted when I was a kid. Spray-painted cars, detailing. I got busted for graffiti a few times."

Tate smiled and nodded. "Ah, so you have a steady hand and you like color."

"I guess."

Tate gestured for Max to take a seat, which he did. "So I have to ask, what do you want to gain from this, Max?"

Max laughed without humor. "For Doc to leave me the fuck alone."

Tate snorted. "I hear ya. But you need to want to do this for it to be of any benefit. I know Dr. Watts arranged this and the reasons why, but I want to know that you're going to give it a chance."

Max scanned around the expansive room, seeing the wooden easels, paintbrushes, color-splattered oilcloths and sheets, and sensed a small lift of exhilaration in his chest. He exhaled. "I want to be able to . . . express myself better. I need to express myself better because I need to *get* better."

Looking back at Tate, he met a beaming grin. "I like it," Tate said gently.

Max smiled. "When do we start?"

●   ●   ●

They started the following day.

Max found that getting out of bed was a little bit easier that morning, despite waking twice with night terrors, and was almost five minutes early to his allotted time. He wouldn't say he was excited per se, but he was certainly looking forward to picking up a paintbrush again. Tate greeted him with a smile, a handshake, and another T-shirt that, beneath a picture of Leonard Nimoy, stated "Spock On." Max considered briefly that maybe Tate needed an appointment with Elliot more than he did.

"I took the liberty of setting an easel up for you," Tate said, leading Max over to a large tripod. "My question for you is, do you want a canvas, or are you starting smaller?"

Max considered his question. He'd never really painted on anything other than brick, concrete, or metal. "Canvas," he replied. "Go big or go home, right?"

Tate slapped his hand against Max's shoulder. "Outstanding."

Set up with his canvas and choice of acrylics, Max perched on a roller stool and thought about what he wanted to say, what he wanted to show. Elliot had told him to express himself, but where the fuck was he supposed to start? The past couple of years had all but drained what inspiration he had dry. The other two guys in the room were busy painting and sketching like lunatics. Max sat for twenty minutes, doing nothing, before Tate approached.

"Okay?" he asked, leaning on his cane. Max shrugged and sipped from his bottle of water. "Tell me, Max, when you used to paint, where were you, who were you with?"

Max's hands found his hair. "In the city or in the body shop with my best friend or my dad."

"Did you have a routine?"

Max's eyebrows met above his nose. "A what?"

Tate lifted his shoulders. "I don't know, like, did you have a particular shirt you wore when you painted, boots, gloves, a particular brush, or product, any music?"

A lightbulb illuminated Max's memories. "My dad always played rock music in the shop, or I had my iPod."

Tate smiled. "Wait there." He limped off quickly, leaving Max perplexed, and returned with an iPod in his hand, out of which hung a pair of white earbuds. "My taste in music probably isn't what you would call rock," Tate admitted. "That's more my brother's style, but if you give me some bands I could put a playlist together for you." He held out the iPod. "Take it. Have a listen, maybe it'll jog something."

Max took the iPod, staring at Tate, as pieces of a jigsaw fell slowly into place in the back of his mind. "Moore," he whispered, once again observing Tate's height, bulk, and familiar smile. He stood quickly. "I'll be goddamned. You're Riley's brother, the doctor, the war hero!"

Tate's cheeks pinked. "I think hero is a bit of a stretch. I prefer black sheep, but, yeah, Riley's my brother. Unless he owes you money and then I'll contest all knowledge and connections."

Max laughed. "Fuck, man." He held out his palm, shaking Tate's hand again. "We never met, you were always away, but I heard a lot about you from Riley. You were in medical school, then Iraq, right?" He glanced at the cane.

"And Afghanistan."

"Wow. Thanks for that, man. I've known Riley nearly ten years. He's babysitting my shop while I'm here. I really don't know what I'd have done without his help, and—"

Tate's smile was all-knowing.

Max pulled his hand back. "But you knew that already."

"Of course. I always research my clients."

"You do?" Max asked dubiously.

"Yeah." Tate looked toward the ceiling. "Plus I called Riley and asked. He said your shop is doing just fine, by the way."

Max chuckled and sat down. "I'm sure there's a rule somewhere about patient confidentiality that you've just admitted to breaking."

Tate waved a flippant hand. "Pfft, patient confidentiality's not even a thing anymore."

Max laughed again. Yeah, he was definitely Riley's brother. He held the iPod tightly. "Thanks for this."

Tate nodded. "My pleasure."

4

Grace Brooks cursed her brother up and down for being so freaking tall.

Seriously, the man was a mountain. And it wasn't because she was bitter being an above-average five foot six; it was because she was struggling to keep her gloved hands over his eyes as she led him down a snow-covered dirt driveway toward the surprise she'd kept secret for nearly a month and a half.

"Look, you made me drive you all the way out here to see whatever it is you want me to see and—" He stumbled. "Are we nearly there?" Kai asked, his posture clearly giving him a hard time. And it wasn't any wonder. He was almost bending completely backward to accommodate his sister's lack of height.

"Yep," Grace replied, pulling to a stop. "Okay. One. Two. Three." She pulled her hands away from Kai's eyes and opened her arms wide. "Ta-da!"

She watched Kai stand to his full height, adjusting the gray scarf around his neck. His dark chocolate eyes narrowed slowly as he took in the two-story house sitting back from the drive, surrounded by dense forest. His silence and the pinch of his mouth made Grace shift from one foot to the other.

"Well," Grace said encouragingly. "Isn't it great?"

His eyebrows lifted at her choice of adjective. He leaned his weight to the right and crossed his arms over his broad chest. "It's definitely something," he commented carefully.

Disappointment bloomed in Grace's stomach.

"I bought it," she continued anyway. "You're always telling me to move on, do something crazy, well . . . here's crazy!"

Kai rubbed a palm across the back of his neck. "I know, I just didn't think it'd be *this* crazy." He gestured toward the house. "Grace, it doesn't even have a front door. Or windows. The roof is barely existent, and it— Wait, is that a toilet on the porch?"

Grace grabbed her brother's forearm, yanking him toward the house, the first thing she'd ever owned in her twenty-six years. "You need to use your imagination. Don't look at what it is now. Think about what it *could* be."

"I don't think even Dr. Seuss would have enough imagination."

Grace huffed, stopping by the termite-ridden porch. "I don't need you to be a sarcastic ass right now, I need you to be fun and un-adult and . . ."

"Imaginative?" Kai smirked.

Grace snapped her fingers. "Yes! Imaginative."

Her brother sniggered and looked up at the house. Surely, Grace thought, he of all people could see the property's potential. Sure, it was run-down and would probably take a million years and a shitload of elbow grease to turn it into something habitable, but it was hers, and that, after everything she'd been through, was something Grace couldn't help but get excited about.

"Obviously," she began, standing straight as she launched into her sales pitch, "in its present condition, it was a steal. I know it'll cost to make it pretty, but that's the fun part. I want to paint it white so it stands out and have a blue door just like Momma's house used to. What do you think?"

Kai opened his mouth but she continued before he could take a breath. "The construction company in town has already taken measurements and my ideas and, holy hell, their plans are amazing. They'll start in the new year, depending on the weather." She pointed toward the upper level. "It has three bedrooms so there's room for you to come and stay whenever you want to hide from your harem of women, and there's also space for an amazing dark-room and, God, Kai, imagine the photographs I could take here!"

She looked from the house to her brother and blinked at his cocked eyebrow. "What?"

"I *don't* have a harem of women."

She snorted. "Kai, I've lived with you in DC for eighteen months; it's like a freakin' carousel of breasts at your place with names like Charissa or Sashina." She elongated the vowel.

"Sasha."

"Whatever."

He laughed and shook his head in disagreement, despite knowing that she was right. Grace wasn't ignorant enough not to see why he had women all but breaking down his front door. Her younger brother was charismatic, intelligent, funny, and a looker. He was also the very best person she knew.

Kai observed her for a moment before leaning closer. "You don't *have* to move out, Grace. I like you living with me. You keep my carousel of breasts in order." She smacked his arm, both of them laughing. His face quickly turned serious. "Are you sure you'll be okay with the distance from DC, getting to your sessions and everything?" He glanced around. "It's pretty remote out here and I'm not sure I like that you're staying in a boardinghouse. I told you, you can stay with me as long as you need."

Grace smiled gratefully. "I know you did, and thank you."

"But?"

Grace shrugged. "But I feel like it's time. I like how remote it is and I'll be okay. I only have sessions every other week now. I don't feel unsafe here. Plus, you'll be over to visit." She looked back at her house, imagining how beautiful it would look when it was finished. "Momma left us that money to do something great. This is what I want."

Kai knocked her shoulder with his. His expression was one she hadn't seen for a very long time. It was soft, satisfied, and, dare she say, impressed. She pulled her ponytail, poking out from under her woolly hat, over her shoulder and started playing with the ends, losing her fingers in the thick black curls.

Kai stilled her hand, recognizing the nervous gesture. "I'm proud of you, sis," he murmured. His eyes hardened distantly. "After he"—Grace's heart stuttered—". . . all *that* happened, I never thought I'd see you excited or passionate about anything. Ever again." He smiled, his teeth shining a beautiful white against his caramel skin, which matched her own. "Seeing you like this is . . . amazing." He looked up at the house. "And, honestly, I think it's *really* great."

* * * *

"So, almost two weeks since your episode. How are you feeling?"

Max knew he'd feel much better if everyone stopped referring to his panic attack as a fucking episode. "Okay," he answered with a lift of his shoulders. "I've checked my blood sugar more, trying to eat right. I paint nearly every day."

Elliot beamed. "Yes, Dr. Moore tells me you've really taken to the art classes." A smile pulled at Max's mouth at his therapist's praise. "Want to tell me about what you've painted?"

The chances were high that Elliot and Tate had already had a powwow about Max's work, but he was prepared to humor him, in spite of the ache in his chest. He took a deep breath and held it. "I was thinking about . . . Chris—Christopher. My son." He reached quickly for the glass of water at the side of his chair and took a huge gulp, praying for it to ease the burning acid creeping up from his stomach.

Elliot remained silent and still, though his eyes were soft and thoughtful.

Christopher had been Max and Lizzie's baby boy, and had inspired the flashes of blue paint that burst from his canvas. A baby who wasn't planned but was loved all the same, inspiring the red and subtle pink circles of tender brushstrokes. A baby who brought him and Lizzie closer than they'd ever been, another reason to stay clean and on the straight and narrow, as he had promised Lizzie he would be so she'd agree to be his alone. A baby who motivated Max to propose to Lizzie, pledging his eternal love to her and their unborn son, with a diamond as big as his heart, knowing that, with the arrival of his son, Max would finally become the man he always wanted to be. A man who would have made his father proud.

Christopher died at the beginning of Lizzie's third trimester.

At almost seven months pregnant, after Lizzie hadn't felt Christopher move or kick for three days, her labor was induced and Max sat at her side while she gave birth to their lifeless son. Lizzie howled. Literally, howled in agony, like an animal. Jesus, he'd never forget that sound for as long as he lived. The grief of Christopher's loss damn near broke her in half. Max had tried to be strong, tried to hold her and tell her it would be okay, but he knew it wouldn't, couldn't. That day something between them, something monumental and vital to their relationship, died, too.

That was the second time Max had thought about taking his own life. The moment he held his minute baby son in his arms— the most exquisite thing he'd ever laid eyes on, eyes closed as though he were simply asleep—he knew that heaven must be the most perfect place, filled with creatures as beautiful as Christopher, a place he'd much rather be.

Lizzie hadn't been able to face seeing the baby. She'd sobbed and screamed until the doctor gave her a sedative to sleep. Despite her eyes opening a day later, Max knew, deep in the cracks of his shattered heart, that she hadn't truly awoken. She was lost to him, too. From that moment, she no longer lived but existed, and Max's sorrow began to overwhelm him.

The funeral was excruciating, another headstone bearing the O'Hare name. The following weeks were worse. For the first time since the night he'd laid eyes on Lizzie, Max threw himself back into the warm and loving arms of his beloved white powder. With Carter in Arthur Kill prison and his friends keeping a distance from Max's volatile, high, or drunk temper, he'd never felt more alone, more lost. Until one particular morning.

That brought Max to the third time he'd wanted to end it all: the morning he woke to find Lizzie gone.

"How did you feel when you realized she wasn't coming back?" Elliot asked.

Max held the most obvious, curse-riddled remark back and pulled his hood closer around his head. "Confused. Angry. Alone . . . Relieved."

Elliot's face didn't change. "Explain relieved to me."

Max closed his eyes, remembering the vacant, grieving, deathly face of the woman he'd loved so fiercely. "I was relieved because I knew I wasn't helping her," he admitted, quietly surprised at the confession. "I was relieved because she took the initiative and left the ruins of us."

"But she left *you*."

Max scoffed. "With the drinking and coke I was doing again? I'd have left, too."

Elliot wrote. "And looking back, thinking about your painting, do you think she made the right choice?"

"I'll never forgive her for walking away without a word," Max spat. "That's what kills me. I earned more than her silence. I was *worth* more. Okay, leave, but we'd been through too much together for her to leave without a good-bye or a fuck-you. We made a child together, for fuck's sake; we were engaged!" Fury rose through Max's body, lighting his blood with disappointment and heartache. "She slunk away like a coward, like she was the only one who hurt, who cried, who missed our son. It was fucking selfish." He sat forward, his elbows resting on his knees, tears scratching at the back of his throat. "But if she got better, moved on after we lost Christopher . . . She made the right choice for her."

Elliot was quiet for so long, Max lifted his head to check whether his therapist was still breathing. He was. "Monday," he murmured. "I'm booking you in with the facility trainer for your first gym session."

Max blinked in surprise. "Okay."

•   •   •

Tate stood behind Max, chewing on the licorice whip Max had shared. "Man," he exclaimed with a satisfied groan. "These things are like fucking crack." He clapped Max's shoulder. "No disrespect."

Max laughed and chewed his own licorice.

"I mean, I haven't had any since I was a kid. And even then Riley would steal them and hide them away." He sighed heavily. "Truthfully, I don't even know why I still speak to him."

Max looked up at his art therapist and grinned at his choice of T-shirt, which stated, "No pants are the best pants," and wondered what seeing the two Moore brothers together would actually be like. In fact, if he remembered correctly, he was pretty sure there were four brothers; he'd met the youngest, Seb, a couple of times. Regardless, Max was certain chaos would ensue.

"I got Dr Pepper, too," he said, waving his red whip. "Carter's a legend."

"Not too shabby," Tate agreed. "He just sent you a care package?"

"And he's coming to visit in the new year." Of course, Max was excited about Carter's visit, but admittedly nervous as hell.

The unexpected but awesome box of sugary delights had arrived the day before, wrapped in Christmas paper with a card from Carter and Kat and signed by all the boys at the body shop—including Riley—wishing him well and a merry Christmas. For a couple of moments it had made Max feel terrific, feel wanted and cared for, but then he'd remembered he was miles away from them all and how much he missed being at home with his friends. The mood swings and claws of anxiety were never far away, no matter how much better he felt. Nevertheless, he'd certainly made a few new friends with the red licorice. And the M&M's.

"So," Tate sang nonchalantly. "Word on the corridor is that you'll be hitting the gym on Monday. Nice."

Max agreed. He couldn't wait to take some latent anger out on some unsuspecting piece of gym equipment.

"I like what you're doing here," Tate added, gesturing to the swirl of soft brown against the black background of Max's second painting. His first was complete and sat in his room in all its terrifying, angry glory. Finishing it didn't curb the underlying anger inside him but, instead, awoke a dormant urge to paint more. It was still early days, but Max was starting to express himself, just as Elliot had asked. And it felt good. Satisfying. Almost as though each brushstroke was quelling some silent hunger inside of him. He was under no illusions; he knew he was purging, all but vomiting his vitriol, addiction, and sorrow onto the canvas—the raw emotion of his first picture was testament to that—but that was okay. If it kept the doctors and staff off his back and the panic attacks at bay, he was more than willing to keep painting.

Tate chewed noisily on his licorice. "The contrast between the colors is nice. What does it mean?"

Max cocked his head, regarding his work. All he knew was that, after his talk with Elliot about Lizzie leaving, he had to get back into the art room and paint . . . something. "Not a clue, dude," he answered, following the diagonal streaks of orange and red with his eyes. He smirked. "You know you shouldn't ask stupid questions."

Tate grinned. "I know. I was just messing with you." He turned with his licorice still hanging from his mouth and approached another painter. Max smiled after him. If nothing else, at least Tate kept him entertained.

5

Max should have known that the easy, lighter sensation that had burrowed within him somewhere along the line of group meetings, talking to Elliot, and painting wouldn't last. The Christmas decorations and luscious food, cheerful music, and presents of socks and chocolate the facility provided caused Max to enjoy the festive period for the first time in years, despite being away from home and familiar faces.

Too bad the warm, let's-love-baby-Jesus fuzzies hadn't stuck around.

Oh, Max O'Hare was, and always had been, a pessimistic bastard on an almost unhealthy scale. And yet, as the days had turned into weeks of his stay in rehab, he'd allowed himself to consider the possibility that he was getting better, that his thoughts were no longer dictated by rage or anguish, and that what had been the regular tap-tapping of addiction in his mind every hour of every day had slowly become a light caress.

Yeah, he'd been a fucking fool.

And the way Elliot was looking at him, that patronizing concerned way of his, was not what he needed in his current mood. But that was what was really pissing him off. He couldn't understand what had him so out of shape, so antsy. He'd battered seven shades of shit out of the gym equipment—earning apprehensive glances from his trainer—and had run on the treadmill until he'd almost collapsed, but the agitation still prickled his skin like nettles.

"You made a phone call this afternoon," Elliot started, gazing at him over the rim of his Phillies mug as he took a sip. "Who did you speak to?"

Max slumped in his seat and drew a large breath. "Carter."

Elliot smiled. "Great. How is he?"

Max's molars ground together. "Engaged." The word shot from him like a bullet from a gun, smothered in hurt, jealousy, and anger. "He's . . . he's fucking engaged." He rubbed his hands down his face, hating the word and hating himself for being such a selfish prick.

The sound of Elliot's mug being placed back onto the side table ricocheted through Max's brain. His tired, addled brain. Fuck. For the first time in four weeks, Max craved a line.

He craved three.

And a bottle of Patrón held by a woman with long legs, great tits, and no morals.

Yeah, he could seriously go for a hot, sweaty, coke-induced fuck to clear his mind.

"You're angry." Elliot didn't pose the question but implied it in the small lift of his hand.

"Yeah," Max barked back without a thought. "No. Goddammit, I don't know what to feel."

Honestly, his head was a cacophony of fucked-up.

He stood from his seat and paced toward the window, which overlooked the vast gardens of the center. The snow was thick and glittered in the afternoon sun. He closed his eyes and leaned his head against the frigid glass. The conversation with Carter had been fine. He'd managed to hide his shock and unacceptable anger at Carter's news. He'd thanked him for the box of treats and they'd shot the shit and joked about Riley's planning of the bachelor party, but it was strained. At least on Max's side.

"I don't know why I feel so—I can't even describe it." It was like a coiled wire around his insides pulling tighter and tighter.

"I understand."

Max turned to his therapist. "You do?"

"Of course. He's your best friend. There's history there. You've seen each other through the hardest parts of your lives and now you're here. His life is moving forward and you feel stagnant."

Max blinked. Well, shit.

"But you're not stagnant, Max," Elliot urged. "The changes I've seen in you in the past couple of weeks have been remarkable. You're opening up."

Max pushed his hands into his pockets. "It doesn't feel that way." With a sigh, he meandered back to his chair and sat down, heavy and weary. He fidgeted under Elliot's unrelenting silence, and tried to hide under his hood. "I want Carter to be happy," he said finally, picking at the cuticle around his thumbnail. "I can't think of anyone who deserves it more."

"Who is he marrying?"

"Kat. They met when he was inside Kill. It's a long story but they also have a lot of history. Saved her life when he was, like, eleven." He laughed without humor. "He's crazy about her, totally fuckin' gaga."

"Like you were with Lizzie."

Max flinched, although the pain he was so used to had numbed considerably. "Yeah, just like that."

Elliot shifted in his seat. "And this is the problem."

"Maybe," Max confessed quietly.

Maybe he was envious that his best friend had found what Max had been so desperate to have. Maybe he was angry that Carter was living his life while he was stuck in East Bumfuck nowhere. Maybe he was a shithead for thinking anything other than congratulations for the man who had always had his back.

"I don't want my past to excuse my resentment. It's shameful," he murmured.

"But you need to handle it instead of pushing it away," Elliot replied. "Deal with the jealousy and move on. When you get home, you can celebrate with him, enjoy his happiness; things will feel different, better."

Max wasn't so sure, but he could hope.

"Besides," Elliot added brightly, "you're young; you could meet someone, fall in love again."

Max's eyes widened while his heart galloped and pounded behind his ribs. "No way," he hissed.

Elliot shrugged, nonplussed. "Why? Life moves on, Max, as Carter is showing. You, too, can have love and joy again."

Max shook his head firmly. "Fuck that. I'm never giving myself to someone like that again. Ever."

It'd kill him for certain.

Besides, all addicts were discouraged from getting involved in romantic relationships in the first twelve months of their recovery. Relationships were too unpredictable and the ups and downs were potential triggers for hitting a luscious Baggie of white powder or a large bottle of Jack. Not that Max could contemplate having a serious relationship ever again. His interactions with women prior to his admittance were fleeting and emotionless. He was a red-blooded male with needs, after all, and his merry-go-round of eager ass was exactly what he needed: detached and simple.

Elliot regarded him thoughtfully before dipping his chin in acknowledgment. "Maybe that's a conversation for another day."

Placing his legal pad on the arm of his chair, he stood and crossed the office toward his elegant bespoke desk. "I have something for you." He opened a drawer, retrieving something from inside. He held out his hand. "Here."

Max lifted from his seat on drowsy legs and approached his therapist. "What?"

Elliot reached for Max's wrist and placed a small round piece of metal into his palm. It took Max a moment to recognize what it was. "It's your first chip, Max. Congratulations. Thirty days clean and counting."

Max stared at the unassuming medallion, punctuated by the "1 Month" in the center and surrounded by words he knew by heart from group: "freedom, goodwill, self, God, society, service."

Jesus, had it really been thirty days since he'd been admitted?

"Thirty-three, actually," Elliot said, as though reading Max's thoughts. Slowly, he placed his hand over Max's, curling their fingers around the chip. His expression was not one of a doctor, but of a friend, kind and reassuring. "With the new year only days away, let this, your determination and strength, prove that happily-ever-afters are achievable, Max. This, right here, is a symbol of hope. It can happen. Even for you."

Max knew the sentiment should have made him all warm and cozy inside, should have backhanded the fear and pessimism out of his head, from around his bruised and scarred heart, and although he was quietly proud that he held his month of struggle away from his friends and all he knew in his palm, he stubbornly shook his head.

"Thank you, but happily-ever-afters don't exist for me, Doc," he said quietly, lifting his head to meet Elliot's stare. "With all the people I've lost in my life, I know that's the real fuckin' truth."

• • •

The bar Grace walked into was not what she expected.

Large windows and a glass door leading out to the back of the place, which would no doubt be incredible in the summer, illuminated the entire space. A fifties-style jukebox played blues, while the pool table and tables and booths of various shapes and sizes filled the rest of the high-ceilinged building. The scent of fries and draft beer clung to every inch of the place, bringing a nostalgic smile to Grace's face.

From the front, the place couldn't look less inviting with its dark wood paneling and faded sign declaring the name to be WHISKEY AND WINGS. During his visit, as they'd strolled past on their way to dinner, Kai had commented about the types of regulars a bar such as Whiskey and Wings would attract, and dragged her away by her elbow before she could do something *else* crazy.

Not to be discouraged, and determined to take control of her life for the first time in years, Grace had decided to embrace the interest in her gut and inquire about the help-wanted sign stuck haphazardly in the corner of the large, grubby window. It had been a while since she'd tended bar, but she'd enjoyed the laughs and the hustle and bustle, even though the job had led her to meet—

"Can I help you, honey?" The West Virginia drawl of the question curled around Grace like a warm hug.

The woman wiping glasses behind the bar was blonde, with a chest that would have every other female in the vicinity standing a little straighter and begging for the number of the store where she'd purchased her push-up. Her lined face was attractive in spite of the heavy-handed mascara and blush. She smiled as Grace approached, and put the glass down.

Grace took a deep breath and removed her woollen hat, her curls bouncing from its clutches. "Hi. I'd like to inquire about the sign."

Blondie leaned the heels of her hands on the edge of the bar and blinked.

Grace swallowed. "The sign asking for help. What are the hours? I only need a couple of shifts a week, but—"

"You're new around here, right?" Her eyes narrowed infinitesimally. Grace was getting used to the suspicious glances and questions expected in a town with a population fewer than ten thousand.

"Yeah. I'm staying at Masen's Boardinghouse," she answered. "I've been in town for—"

"You worked a bar before?"

"Um, yes. It's been a while, but I tended when I was in college and my brother owns a bar in DC, which—"

"Be here on Monday, six thirty sharp."

Grace blanched. "That's— Monday is New Year's Eve."

Blink. "You got plans?"

No, but common sense knew that the place would be jammed. Filled with strangers.

Anxiety whispered over Grace's chest. "I . . . no, that's fine."

"Good. I don't know what shifts I'll need you for after that, maybe every other day or night, maybe not, I need you to be flexible, but I sure as hell will need you Monday." Deep blue eyes traveled down Grace's body, taking in her winter boots, jeans, gloves, and thick jacket with a wry smile. "And wear something pretty."

Grace looked down at herself. "Okay."

"Knock it off, Holly." A deep male voice came from the doorway. "She already looks pretty."

The man was dressed in a police uniform: a dark shirt, tie, and khaki pants. He was tall and lean with wavy auburn hair and a well-groomed goatee that lifted when he smiled at her. He watched her for a beat before stepping forward with his hand out. "I'm Deputy Sheriff Caleb Yates. I don't think I've had the pleasure."

Grace swallowed, nervous butterflies swarming her stomach. Ridiculous, she chastised herself. He's a police officer. He's no threat. And his blue eyes were safe and honest. She breathed deeply and smiled back, shaking his large hand. "I'm New-In-Town Grace Brooks."

He laughed politely at her lame joke. "I've heard. You've caused quite a stir around here. We don't get many new faces that stay longer than a vacation here in Preston County. You've bought the Baileys' old place, right?"

He knew a lot, which immediately put Grace on edge. She fisted her hands together while her eyes darted past him toward the exit. The deputy badge on the left side of his chest knocked her around the head with a dose of calm-the-hell-down. Of course he knew about the house; he probably knew everyone's business. That was his job.

"I have, yes," she confirmed, not wanting to say anything more, uncomfortable under the two pairs of scrutinizing eyes.

Caleb rocked on his heels, crossing his arms over his chest. "That's great. It's about time someone tackled that behemoth of a building."

Grace laughed shortly. "Well, I'm your girl." The sparkle in the deputy's almond-shaped blues was flattering but had Grace's feet moving around him. "Anyway, I'd better get back. Thanks . . . Holly. I'll be here on Monday."

She waved a shaking hand over her shoulder, ignoring whatever Holly's reply was, and all but stumbled out of the door onto the snow-covered street. Hurrying down the sidewalk as best as she could with the cold taunting the old injuries to her right hip and rib cage, she stopped inside the mouth of a small alleyway and pressed her back against the damp brick.

Leaning her head back, Grace breathed as slowly and as deeply as she could, fighting the fear back with the cold, fresh West Virginia air and the fact that her past was thousands of miles away on the other side of the country, on parole with a court-issued restraining order and her old apartment. Her throat narrowed as his face flickered behind her eyelids.

Maybe Kai was right. Maybe this wasn't such a great idea. Maybe it *was* too soon for her to be out alone, out in a strange place. Maybe she *wasn't* strong enough to be around unfamiliar people yet. Maybe she should pack up, forget the old house, and head back to DC.

"No," she croaked toward the freezing sky. She wasn't giving up that easy. These moments were bound to happen; she just had to fight through them. Her breathing slowed. She opened her eyes, hating the tears that filled them. "Great," she whispered, pulling her hat back on. Now the deputy and her new boss would think she was a raving loony after she'd behaved so rudely.

Well, as her momma used to say, what's done is done. Grace knew she'd simply have to show them that she wasn't a complete weirdo when she went to work on Monday. Her pulse jumped, this time in excitement. A job. It might be for only a few hours a week but she had an actual job. Kai would shit bricks. She laughed to herself, thinking of the conversation they would no doubt have that evening when she called to tell him, and slowly left the safety of her alleyway, heading back to the boardinghouse.

Yes, the dark clouds of her past continued to follow her daily, but with the house, and now a job, at least they now had beautiful silver linings.

6

Between the painting, the gym visits—which were having an awesome effect on his arms, chest, and waistline—group sessions, and chats with Elliot, time started to speed up for Max. Days passed in a blur of talking, running, punching, and acrylic paint until, one brisk January afternoon, he received his second medallion. Sixty-four days of clean living and, Max had to admit, he was feeling pretty good. He'd even quit smoking.

He'd built up a solid friendship with Tate and always looked forward to their sessions, while—although he still wasn't singing like a canary—his therapy with Elliot was also becoming less of a hindrance. He'd spoken more about Lizzie, more about his addiction and the roots of it, not that it would have taken a genius to figure out, and had even allowed himself to consider the future, his time away from rehab.

His stay was never given a time limit, though Elliot had suggested he look to staying another month. He was pleased with Max's progress but wanted Max to be happy and ready to deal with the real world again. The after-care program was second to none and Max would obviously have access to sponsors and therapists for as long as he needed, but Max had agreed.

He wasn't ready quite yet.

In truth, the thought of going home—as awesome as it would be—filled Max with an odd sense of trepidation. He was busy every day in the facility, surrounded by people he had grown to recognize and, in many cases, like. Despite the latter being true, Max worried about how he would fill his time when he was home, how he'd move from one day to the next without the rigorous timetable he lived by. Busyness was his new friend. Without it, back home, he'd have a lot of time on his hands; time to ruminate, agonize, wonder where he could get a line.

He was concerned that his friends wouldn't understand, wouldn't recognize how hard Max battled to make it through every day without stuffing that poison up his nose. He knew they'd be supportive, of course; they always had been; but would that be enough? Elliot explained that his fears were understandable and very normal, but still Max fretted.

The reflection that looked back at him in the main hall window showed a much healthier face, though still weathered with lines of struggle. His brown hair had grown into disarray and he hadn't shaved in a couple of days. His dark eyes watched the driveway like a hawk.

"You got a visitor today?"

Max startled at the voice at his side. He turned to see Dom, from his group session, peering out of the window, too. Max nodded. "My best friend." He turned back to the window. "It's the first time I've seen him since he left me here." He swallowed. No, that wasn't fair. "Actually, he helped me get in here. Paid for everything."

"Awesome," Dom commented, always a man of few words. Max noticed how much better the man looked, too, in comparison to when they'd first been introduced, and wasn't that a strange thought? Two men, two addictions, but both with the same goal: get clean or get dead.

The two men heard the car before they saw it. The unmistakable roar of a Maserati GranTurismo MC Stradale echoed through the rural surroundings.

"Jesus," Dom muttered as they watched the matte black vehicle pull up to the front of the facility. "Nice wheels."

Max snorted. He just knew Carter would have loved every

minute of driving that damned thing from New York. Boy had always had good taste in automobiles and now that Carter was CEO of the business that was his birthright, he certainly had the money to indulge.

Max and Carter had grown up from small boys watching and working in Max's father's body shop, where they'd learned what the term "muscle car" truly meant, pulling engines apart, and building them back up. They passed their tests and crashed their first cars together, bought motorcycles together, and attended every gearhead event in the continental United States.

They were great times, and as Max watched Carter unfold himself out of the car, he realized how much he'd missed his best friend. They'd been through so much together. So many times, when any normal friendship would have been ripped apart at the seams, the two of them fought yet stayed obstinately loyal to each other. Carter's going to prison in Max's place more than three years ago—so Max could be with Lizzie while she was pregnant instead of doing time for something he didn't do—was just one thing on a long list of shit that Max owed his friend for dearly, and Max was determined, once he was back in the real world, to spend every day paying Carter back.

Despite his initial shock and the dregs of cheap jealousy that still sloshed through him, Max couldn't have been more proud of his best friend. He was happy, healthy, and in love, looking for all the world like the weight of doubt and abandonment he'd always carried around with him since they were kids had at last been shucked off. Max realized with a jolt that Carter had finally found his place in the world, and the slow spread of relief that followed was more than a little welcome.

Carter smiled as Max approached, but it was uncertain, careful, and Max hated it. He knew today was going to be awkward as shit, both Tate and Elliot had warned him, but Max had hoped it wouldn't be.

"Sorry I'm a little late," Carter began, throwing a thumb over his shoulder. "I had to check in with the front desk."

Max shook his head. "It's okay." He stopped two feet from Carter, his hands pushed deep into his pockets, and tilted his chin toward the Maserati. "Compensating for something?"

Carter barked a laugh and lifted his eyebrows, glancing back at the car. "She needed her legs stretching, what can I say?"

"She's beautiful. V-eight?"

"Zero to sixty in four-point-five seconds." Carter nodded with a wry smile. "It would've been rude not to, right?"

Both men chuckled nervously. Max rocked uncomfortably on his heels before reaching out a hand. "It's good to see you, man. Thanks for coming."

Carter pushed his keys into his back pocket and took Max's hand, shaking it first then squeezing before he let go. "Of course. I wouldn't have missed it. Thank you for inviting me. You look . . . well. Better. Much better."

Max couldn't deny that he had the overwhelming urge to hug his friend, because damn it was good to see him, but instead he gestured with his hand toward the path he knew wound its way around the entire facility. "I want to show you around before you meet everyone. Wanna take a walk?"

Carter cleared his throat. "Sure."

Side by side, they walked through the melting snow, as Max pointed through the large windows telling Carter about the art room and his paintings, his group sessions and his meetings with Elliot. It was strange explaining it all, but Max didn't feel the embarrassment that had curled in his stomach the first time he and Carter had spoken on the phone. Seeing him while they spoke was certainly easier.

"Riley told me about Tate working here," Carter said as he peered into the art room where Tate was teaching a class. "Small world, huh? I think I spoke to him on the phone briefly once, but I never met him. Is he as nuts as Riley?"

Max grinned. "Crazy T-shirts aside? He's like Riley, but a little more sane. See the cane? He was injured as a medic on tour with the Marines."

"Yeah, I remember that. It was the only time Riley ever left New York back then."

"Tate hit the pills and painkillers hard when he was honorably discharged from the corps. It was all to do with his injury. Dude picked himself up, went to rehab, went back to school to train as a counselor, and here he is, four years clean and helping other addicts."

Carter smiled. "Sounds like a great guy."

"He is," Max agreed. "He's offered to be my sponsor when I . . . when I come home." Unease swirled tightly in Max's stomach.

Carter's face, however, lit up. "When do you think that'll be?"

Max shrugged. "I just got my two-month medallion, so—"

"That's amazing, brother," Carter uttered, pride and relief prevalent in his voice.

Max held out the two chips in his palm. He carried them everywhere as addicts were encouraged to do, just in case the craving surpassed discomfort; a reminder, a tangible way of counting off the days of his servitude to addiction.

Carter gazed at them, not touching, and smiled. "I knew you could do it."

"Well," Max said slowly, closing his fist around them, "I'm not there yet. Elliot thinks I should stay another month or so."

Carter's brow furrowed. "And how do you feel about that?"

Max put the medallions away and began walking, not able to stomach what would no doubt be a look of disappointment on Carter's face. "I . . . think I need it," he confessed. "I think I still have a lot I need to work out about . . . Lizzie, Christopher—all of the shit that's happened. I'm still not— I can't just forget. I'm trying, Carter, but it's not an overnight thing and I have to live with this shit over me every day when I leave here and—"

Carter's hand on Max's arm made him stop and turn. "Hey, man, it's okay," he murmured, his eyes sad but imploring. "Seriously, buddy, take all the time you need. We'll all be waiting for you when you come home. I don't care how long it takes. We all just want you to get better. *I* want you to get better."

Max exhaled and rubbed a hand down his face. He kicked at a lump of stubborn, unmelted snow and allowed Carter's words of reassurance to calm the disquiet in his chest. "Thanks."

They continued walking around the center. Conversation, although not stilted, felt different. Carter spoke about Kat and, although there was caution in his words, about his proposal to her. Max smiled as best as he could while Carter waxed lyrical about his Peaches, and Carter responded in kind when Max spoke fleetingly about his sessions with Elliot.

The two of them were a fucking nightmare for sure, both of them uncertain because of the weirdness Max's stay in rehab had brought to their friendship. Max could only hope that, when he finally did go home, things would be easier. He could only imagine how hard it was for his best friend. Carter had seen Max at his very worst, when he hit rock bottom, half-naked, unconscious, and unresponsive on the bathroom floor. Max had known Carter nearly his whole life and knew he'd have torn himself to shreds over it all, blamed himself, which was absurd. Max had no one to blame but himself.

And maybe Lizzie.

But he was working on that blame every day.

As part of Max's twelve steps, he'd been urged to acknowledge what his addiction had done to the people he cared for, the people who had tried for so long to help him. Christ, Carter had tried so hard, pushed Max to get better, even when Kat had asked him to step away and let Max do what he wanted; even when—in a moment of insanity—Max had pointed a loaded gun at Carter's head, he'd not lost hope, imploring Max to get the help he so desperately needed—

"Thanks, Carter," Max said before he could even recognize the need to say the words of gratitude.

Seated in the visitors' room with the winter sun streaming through the tall windows, the words reverberated around him. Carter, who'd been chatting amiably with Elliot, turned. He opened his mouth to speak, but Max continued, muttering toward the cup of coffee in his hands. "And I'm sorry for everything I put you through, you *and* Kat—I know you two argued a lot about me, and for that I apologize. I'm sorry for what my addiction put you through and I thank you for being there and not giving up on me. It would have been so easy, but you didn't."

He lifted his head slowly, noticing first the wide smile on Elliot's face. Bastard looked like a proud father seeing his son take his first steps. Almost the literal truth, the words pushed Max stumbling into new territory.

The expression on Carter's face was surprised yet warm, while his eyes suddenly looked a little glassy. He dipped his chin and cleared his throat. "No problem. I've got your back."

Yeah, he always had, and words could never convey how much Max appreciated it.

After a couple of hours during which Carter finally met Tate, fussed over Max's paintings, and saw the rest of the place, Max walked Carter back to his car, feeling lighter, less anxious.

Carter pressed the key fob, making the blinkers of the Maserati flash. "You know," he started, with a deep breath, "when you decide you're ready to come home, you're more than welcome to stay with Kat and me." His words were quick, almost falling over one another. "You could stay with us at the beach house in the Hamptons, away from the city. You could relax, take it slowly. Riley has the body shop under control. The place is back in the black and busy, so you don't need to rush back there until you're ready." He lifted his shoulders. "Staying with us might be better than going back to your empty apartment. At least you wouldn't be alone all the time."

Max smiled gently, curious as to whether Kat had had any say in Carter's offer, or if she even knew of it. "I appreciate that. It sounds good."

Carter smiled. "Well, the offer's there, bud. You let me know."

Max nodded and stepped back as Carter opened his car door and got in. The V-8 engine thundered to life, making the two men sigh with appreciation and lust.

"I'll be driving this baby when I get back," Max taunted as Carter shut the car door and rolled down the window.

"In your wettest and wildest, my friend," Carter retorted, pressing his foot to the gas, making the car purr. Max's laugh was halted by Carter's next words: "I know you can do this, Max." His face was honest and hopeful. "I know it's been strange today and I'm sorry. You have a long way to go, shit to get through about Lizzie and . . . but I know you'll do it. I fucking know it."

Max gripped Carter's shoulder through the car window and squeezed. "Thank you, brother."

7

The apartment was dark when Max staggered through the front door, cursing as his shin smacked into the fucking coffee table that Lizzie had been more than insistent on buying when they first moved in. It was the feature of the room, apparently. Now it just created bruises.

He mumbled to himself about being quiet, chuckling as the buzz of his last few lines lit his veins, making his skin warm and his brain pulse. It had been a crazy night filled with strobe lights, powder, and dancing. The scent of sweat permeated his shirt while the hair on the nape of his neck clung to his skin in soaked clumps. The side of his face throbbed from his chin to his eye socket where some asshole had punched him at the bar. Max had made a jibe about the dude's jacket, and then, when the guy didn't retaliate, Max had commented on the prick's girlfriend. And then—because it was a day ending in y, and Max wanted a fight and a rush of adrenaline to combat the emptiness that spread through his body like the cancer that killed his father—he'd brought up the guy's mother, whom Max didn't know but didn't hesitate to call a complete whore.

There was dried blood on Max's shirtsleeve. Oh, yeah. His nose got busted, too, before his friend Paul had grabbed him by the scruff of the neck and shoved him into a waiting cab just as the night was filled with police sirens and blue flashing lights.

Max sniffed and wiped at his nostrils drunkenly. His nose hurt but as long as he could still breathe through it, he'd lose himself in as much blow as he could if it meant the pain of living would disappear. Fuck, he just wanted to be numb. He wanted to forget. He wanted to pretend that instead of the broken woman he knew he would find in his bed, he'd find the feisty, sparkling creature he'd fallen in love with. Instead of the shut door that concealed all the baby shit they'd bought that neither of them could bear to look at, he wanted to find it wide open, his son healthy and asleep in the white crib . . .

He snorted the back of his hand, desperate for any trace of powder before he pushed the bedroom door open.

Lizzie was exactly where he'd left her, curled up in a ball, unwashed, silent, and fractured by her grief. Max could barely look at her. He wanted to. God, how he wanted to. He wanted to take her in his arms, cleanse her of her pain, and lose himself inside her. He'd make love to her, kiss her fiercely, because kissing her was his favorite thing in the world, and make her forget; make himself forget. But she wouldn't let him near her. She wouldn't speak to him.

And he missed her. He missed her so fucking much.

Stumbling around the room, he managed to undress himself and slide into the bed next to her, desperate to take her into his arms and press himself into the warmth of her skin. Despite the mere inches between their bodies, they'd never been more apart. Max stretched out his fingers, the tips of them dancing lightly over the bare skin of Lizzie's arm. He knew what that part of her body tasted like. He knew what every part of her body tasted like even though it had been months since they'd been together that way. Max understood. At least he tried to, but if she wouldn't listen to his words of love, maybe he could show her what she meant to him with his body.

Before he had the chance to consider her reaction, if he were to roll her over, kiss her, taste her mouth, and thrive off the intimacy he craved from her lips, she pulled her arm away.

"Don't," she croaked. "You stink of beer and you're high again."

He snapped, the buzz loosening his tongue and shortening his temper. "Yeah. Well, shit, I have to get my kicks somehow, right? At least one of us is living."

She sighed, her shoulders rounding away from him even more. "This isn't living, Max. This isn't living."

"What do you want from me, Liz?" he asked, dropping his hand to the mattress, away from her body. "Tell me what the fuck I can do and I'll do it. For fuck's sake talk to me!"

But she didn't. She never did. Instead she locked him out, pulled the covers around her small, fragile body, and shuffled from the bed to the living room, where she resumed her desolate silence on the couch. Max wasn't sure which was worse: having her in bed next to him and not speaking, or her being in the other room. Either way he knew he was losing her. Shit, he'd already lost her, and he had no idea how to get her back.

Hours later, when the dawn light filtered through a small gap in the drapes, waking Max from a broken slumber, he would wonder how he hadn't heard her leave. For days, weeks, months, and years, he would torture himself about how he should have followed her into the living room; done more and pushed her further to open up to him, to share her grief with him.

Even before he skidded down the hallway and saw that her keys, shoes, purse, and coat were gone, he knew she'd left. Even as he hunted through her closet searching for a clue as to where the fuck she might have gone, and relentlessly dialed her cell phone number, and the cell phone numbers of her family and friends, he knew she didn't want to be found. And when he collapsed on the bedroom floor, calling out her name through racking sobs, he knew his heart had been broken forever.

• • •

Max twirled the three-month medallion—ninety-seven days clean—in the palm of his hand. He fidgeted and kicked a foot against his packed bag, avoiding looking directly at either Elliot or Tate, who flanked him as they waited for Carter to arrive.

"So, you've got all your paperwork, my number, your prescription, dates of your first meetings with—"

Max smirked and cocked an eyebrow at Elliot. "Yes, Doc. I have them. Just like I had them the first three times you asked."

Tate snickered into the back of his hand. His T-shirt today was bright green and declared "Warning: If zombies chase us, I'm tripping you." Max chuckled and shook his head. Truthfully, he was going to miss seeing those damned T-shirts every day. Tate was now officially Max's sponsor and the two of them would no doubt see each other a lot, what with meetings and such, but it wouldn't be the same. Max's laugh had definitely been throaty when Tate had given him his own ludicrously inappropriate T-shirt, which stated "Pugs not drugs" under a hoodie-wearing dog.

"As part of your tutelage under me," Tate had deadpanned, "you must wear this at all times." Max was certain having Tate as a sponsor was never going to be boring.

Carter pulled up five minutes later in a red Shelby GT. It was gorgeous and, Max had to admit, ten times nicer than the Maserati. Carter all but leaped out of the car, wide smile of pride front and center. The four of them put Max's bags and paintings into the trunk. Once done, Carter shook both Elliot's and Tate's hands and made himself scarce, silently acknowledging Max's need for privacy.

Max cleared his throat and blinked at his therapist. "Thanks, Doc," he managed. "For everything." He held out his hand, which Elliot shook with a wry smile. Despite their rocky start, Max knew that, without Elliot, he'd never have gotten through the first month, let alone the following two. He'd never admit it aloud, but he was more than thankful that it had been Elliot's office he'd found himself in that very first day.

"This isn't the end," Elliot murmured. "It's just the beginning. You're so much stronger than you give yourself credit for, Max. Never forget that. And there's hope. In all things. The hardest part is done." As hokey as he sounded, Max nodded in understanding. "Dr. Moir is exceptional. He's a great friend of mine and he'll absolutely help you move forward. Nevertheless, you know where I am if you want to talk."

And with that, Elliot made his way back into the center.

"So you've got my cell, my pager, my home number, give me a call whenever, no matter what time, right?" Tate said, a rare moment of seriousness adorning his face. "We'll have our scheduled meet-ups, or whenever you need me. Always. You're not alone."

Max nodded. "I got it."

"And keep painting," Tate implored. "Please. Dude, you have too much talent to stop now. Your work is exceptional. Even if you do it on your downtime. It'll keep your mind busy and away from thinking about—"

"I got it."

Tate smiled. "Good." He sighed. "So we gonna hug this shit out, or what?"

"Thank you," Max said earnestly as they hugged, giving each other an obligatory backslap.

"No problem." Tate released him and grinned, leaning on his cane. "I'll see you soon. Say hello to that asshole brother of mine for me, huh?"

With heavy, chaotic sensations of fear, relief, joy, and sadness filling him from toe to crown, Max saluted Tate once more and climbed into the car. He exhaled heavily and put on his seat belt. Carter sat in silence for a beat before he turned the key in the ignition.

"You okay?" he asked.

Max took in the surroundings of his adopted home one last time and swallowed. He couldn't quite comprehend that he was going back out into the world, away from the safety of his routine and the relationships he'd built. His stay in Pennsylvania had been difficult, to say the least, reflecting on his past, his heartache, and his losses, but without it, Max knew, he'd have eventually become just another headstone on his family's plot, way before his time.

As hard as it was going to be heading back, he finally understood that he couldn't let that happen. His twelve steps urged him to recognize all he had to live for. And he had. Even if it was simply by painting, lifting weights and running, or working back in his body shop, he'd been handed a tiny speck of optimism, and he would cling to it with everything he had. He would focus on moving forward one day at a time. One big-ass foot in front of the other.

Elliot's words echoed around his head. *It's just the beginning.*

"Yeah," Max answered before turning to his best friend. He stroked the medallions in his pocket. "I'm okay."

8

Carter's beach house in the Hamptons was just as beautiful as Max remembered despite the falling rain and the wind that whipped around them, as he and Carter trudged up the deck steps to the front door. Inside, a fire flickered in the hearth, and the guest room Carter led him to was made up as though they were expecting the sultan of Brunei. Towels, flat-screen TV, bamboo blinds at the windows, huge comforter, and fluffy pillows, soft-looking rug on the floor, and, wait, a vanity set?

Carter clapped his hands together. "Okay. So, I'm thinking fuck it, let's have pizza for dinner."

Max's stomach growled. "Awesome," he replied, kicking off his sneakers and dropping onto the edge of the bed. He allowed his socked feet to wander onto the rug. Yep, that shit was soft as a baby's ass. He glanced around the room. "This is nice, man."

Carter crossed his arms over his chest. "Yeah, Kat wanted it to be perfect for when you got here. She went a little crazy in Home Depot. I couldn't reel her in." He eyed the fluffy white towels and bathrobe suspiciously. "Sorry."

Max tried to hide his surprise with a chuckle. "Will she be joining us for dinner?"

Carter shook his head. "Nah, brother. It's just you and I tonight. She's staying in the city. It's easier for her with work. However, I, being the boss, get the day off tomorrow."

Max snorted and fell back on the bed. "Fucking slacker."

"Blow me," Carter retorted, walking out of the room. "I'll go and order dinner before I set up *COD* on the Xbox," he called from the top of the stairs.

Max smirked toward the ceiling.

Yeah, shit between them was going to be just fine.

.   .   .

With bellies full of the best pizza ever and after thoroughly whipping Carter's ass on the Xbox, Max followed him down to the house's converted basement. A hybrid man cave and gym, Carter called it, separated by a wall through the middle of the space. Max marveled at the gym equipment Carter had acquired on one side and the full-size pool table, jukebox, sofas, and bar on the other.

"You wanna break?" Carter asked as he set up the table, gesturing with his hand toward the cues lined up against the wall.

For two hours, Max and Carter caught up. Without the pressure of the rehab center around them and without anyone else around to interrupt, their conversation flowed just as easily as the Diet Coke and Oreos, which Carter pulled from a small secret cupboard under the bar.

"You can't tell Kat about this stash," Carter said with mock seriousness.

"I'll take it to the grave," Max promised, stuffing another cookie into his mouth. "I'll definitely need to use your gym shit." He patted his stomach.

"Feel free to use what you want," Carter insisted, lining up a shot and pocketing a ball in the top right. "There's space in here and your room if you want to do some painting, too." Max didn't reply, too overwhelmed with gratitude to speak. Carter stood up straight from the table, worry etching his brow. "That's if you want to, man. I don't know. You should."

Max nodded. "I want to. It's just . . ." Carter stood still, silent. "The painting thing was weird. Doc wanted me to do it, bribed me, in fact. Bastard. Tate encouraged me. I knew I wanted to try it again, knew I had to express myself, as Doc put it, and when I picked up the brush it was like . . . I just purged, ya know? All the hate, anger, and all of me that's been a fucking mess for so long, just spewed onto the canvas. Some bits I don't even remember doing."

"Did it help?"

Max took a deep breath, recollecting the satisfaction of when he saw his first painting completed, the weight that lifted slowly with each brushstroke, and how it helped him open up more with Elliot and group. "Yeah," he replied. "It helped."

Carter smiled gently. "Then do it."

* * * *

"Well, I'll be goddamned, if it isn't Max O'Hare!" Riley Moore's voice boomed across the body shop, reverberating around the metal and the people working on it.

Max laughed and lost himself in the huge man-hug Riley embraced him with. Riley clapped Max's cheek. "You're looking good, my man. My brother Tate knows his shit, right?"

Max snorted. "Yeah, he knows his shit."

All the other boys—Paul, Cam, and a couple of faces Max didn't recognize—all approached him with handshakes, hugs, and well wishes. It had been a week since he'd left rehab but it was the first time he'd been back into the city and visited his business. He was relieved but not surprised that the place looked great and ridiculously busy. He noted a small blonde-haired woman at the back of the shop, sitting behind a desk working on a pile of paperwork, oblivious to the hubbub of Max's arrival, and shook his head wryly. Carter had told him all about the young, pretty thing Riley had "welcomed" into the world of O'Hare's.

He pushed Riley's shoulder. "You never fucking change."

Riley smirked. "What? I gots needs."

"You sure everything's good?" Max hedged, glancing around the place, a strange sensation of neutrality settling in his belly.

"Absolutely," Riley answered, his business face emerging quickly. "We don't have the figures for the last quarter here, although Carter might at WCS, but you're obviously welcome to look at the books if you want—"

Max clapped a hand to Riley's shoulder and smiled. "No need. I trust you. And I can't thank you enough." He lowered his voice slightly. "Carter showed you my offer, right?"

Max couldn't have been certain, but Riley appeared almost shy, certainly grateful, his hazel eyes soft. "Yeah, man, he did. It's fantastic. Thank you."

Max and Carter had discussed at length making Riley a permanent business fixture at the body shop. With Carter's company, WCS, becoming a shareholder in O'Hares, clearing all the debts when Max first entered rehab, and Riley's business know-how in maintaining the smooth running of the place in Max's absence, it seemed only appropriate to offer Riley a firmer stake in the place, as well as a salary. Besides having good and trusted friends at the helm of his beloved father's business, Max also knew that, for a time, he could afford to take a step back, take his time in finding his feet again in the outside world, reducing by a considerable amount the weight of the expectations that rested on his shoulders.

Catching up with the guys at the shop was a strange experience. They all looked happy to see him, especially Paul, who, like Carter, had begged Max to get help for months, if not years, before he finally went to rehab. But Max couldn't shake the feeling of detachment that had continually skulked within him over the past seven days.

He'd been eagerly filling his time at Carter's beach house with the treadmill—when the weather wasn't agreeable enough for him to run on the beach—weights, playing guitar, reading, and even painting a little, but the ball of restiveness still weighed heavy in his spine. He'd continued to take his meds regularly, exactly when he should; attended his first NA meeting outside of rehab; spoken to Tate about it and arranged his first appointment with Dr. Moir; but still Max couldn't settle.

Carter had done more than bend over backward to accommodate Max's needs, making sure that he had everything he could want to make his transition back into the real world as easy as possible. Kat, too, had been supersweet, cooking for the three of them and appearing genuinely interested in Max's recovery. She didn't cling to Carter, as Max had assumed she might now that Max was back. She was, as always, attractive, ballsy, and independent. Even in the short time Max had spent with her and Carter in their home, it was still abundantly clear why they worked well together, even if the diamond on her left hand still caused Max's stomach to twist in residual grief.

It was all very bizarre and difficult to digest.

"You'll get there," Tate assured him on the phone when they spoke later that evening, as Max lazed on the bed in Carter's guest room.

"Maybe I should go home," he mused, although the sound of the ocean certainly kept him calmer than the noise of Brooklyn. "Maybe being in my own apartment might help?"

"If you think it will, do it," Tate encouraged. "But don't isolate yourself."

Max sighed and rubbed his face with a tired hand. "Yeah. Christ, I just didn't think it would be so . . ."

"Different."

"Yeah," Max agreed enthusiastically. "Everyone is being so fucking nice, so happy for me to be home, despite the shit I put them all through, but I just can't . . . connect or relax."

"Ants in your pants?"

"I guess. And I'm trying to keep busy and do things that keep my mind occupied. I want everything to go back to . . . before. Truth is, I've not stopped since I got back." And he was tired, emotionally and physically. As nice as it was seeing all the familiar faces of his friends, it unnerved a deep-rooted part of Max. A part he hadn't realized existed. These people, despite their smiles, were people he'd hurt, fucked over, disappointed, and even partied with.

Tate sighed. "A common mistake people can make once they get home is that they try to take on too much right away. You can't fix all the problems in your life in one week, Max. The first couple of years of recovery are a time of recuperation. You're still fragile, man."

The word made Max's molars grind, but he understood Tate wasn't trying to patronize him. Parts of him would continue to be very fragile. He'd come a long way in Pennsylvania, but he would always be a tiny tap away from shattering again. That was the life of an addict. All he could do was stay away from anything and anyone that could cause the damage.

"Take it day at a time," Tate repeated softly. "That's all you can do."

.   .   .

"This place looks incredible!"

Grace couldn't hold back the squee of excitement that burst from her mouth as Kai walked through the downstairs of her no-longer-dilapidated house. It was still a long way from habitable, but with a freak week of dry weather, the builders had—once the termite problem was handled—built a brand-new roof, installed new floors and walls downstairs, and begun constructing the wide stairway up to the first level.

"Can you see it now?" she asked knowingly.

Kai laughed and tapped a palm against one of the new walls. "I can. I doubted I would, but I can."

Grace fist-bumped the air.

"The work is really good, too," Kai commented. "I'm impressed."

"Of course it's good," Grace retorted with an eye roll. "I wouldn't hire just anybody. I'm not entirely helpless, you know. I can make good decisions."

Kai cocked an eyebrow and Grace immediately knew what was coming.

"Don't start," she warned.

The words exploded out of her brother in an incredulous blast. "Working behind a bar, Grace? With your anxiety the way it is. Really? Did you even give it a minute's thought? Working in a place filled with strangers. *Drunken* strangers! The same environment where you met that piece of fuck—"

"Kai." Grace grumbled something offensive under her breath, turned heel, and stormed out of the house into the cool early spring air. "Why can't you just . . ."

Kai's heavy footsteps followed her quickly.

"This has nothing to do with him," she hissed, still marching away from him. "I wanted to see if I could step out of my comfort zone, and I'm pretty sure in the few months I've worked at Whiskey's I've done that. I've not had any attacks or flashbacks—"

"Yes," Kai agreed, still exasperated, almost falling over her when Grace came to an abrupt halt. "But you were told you needed to take things slowly"—he threw an arm back toward the house—"one crazy decision at a time."

"Don't patronize me, Kai," she fumed.

Kai's face dropped minutely, her words clearly surprising him. "That's not my intention, Grace." He pushed his hands into his pockets. "I just— I worry about you. I want to make sure you're safe and I can't do that with you so far away. After what he did to you . . ."

The anger boiling in Grace's blood cooled considerably as she watched her baby brother's shoulders slump in dejection. "I'm all right," she murmured, placing her hand on his forearm and squeezing. "I know you think differently, and I love you dearly for it, but it's not your place to protect me, Kai. Besides, he's a long way away and I'm fine. Really. Sure, I still get nervous, jumpy, but I deal with it. Everyone has been so nice to me."

"Especially Deputy Colin, I'm sure," Kai remarked icily.

Grace snorted and shook her head. "It's Deputy Caleb and he's harmless."

"He looks at you in a way that suggests otherwise, Grace."

Despite the shiver of unease that slipped across her chest, Grace shrugged. "I can handle him. He knows I'm not interested in anything but being friends."

Kai watched her carefully. "Now that you're here doing all of this, do you think you'd ever do that, like . . . *be* with anyone again?"

Grace swallowed and took a deep breath. "I don't know."

The thought of being with a man in an intimate capacity made goose bumps erupt all over her body in alarm, but she couldn't deny the loneliness that tugged at her heart whenever she saw couples in love, happy. Could she ever go there again? Maybe. If she could trust. Would it terrify her? Absolutely. But she'd always been a romantic at heart. It was ingrained in her in spite of what she'd been through at the hands of a man who'd sworn to honor and protect her.

Kai wrapped a strong arm around her shoulders and pulled her close, knowing where her mind had gone. "Come on," he said, kissing her forehead. "You can show me your awesome bar skills and buy me a beer while Deputy Calvin pretends not to drool all over you."

Grace couldn't help but laugh.

9

Sweating like a bitch in heat, Max lumbered into the kitchen of Carter's beach house and headed straight for the fridge. He pulled out a large bottle of water, which he proceeded to gulp. His run down the beach had been exactly what he'd needed after he'd awoken that morning with a hunger for a gram that almost crippled him. The night terrors had come back with a vengeance the previous night, too; a continual loop of images, which had Max fighting with his pillows and sobbing at two in the morning. It was the first time he'd suffered such cravings and nightmares in the three weeks he'd been home and it had done more than shake him.

Tate had been a lifesaver at the end of the phone, offering to drive out, listening and telling him everything he needed to hear. The run had been his idea and Max had thrown himself into it. His body ached deliciously, subduing the craving from a crashing wave to a firm ripple, though the tiredness from his brain's incapability to shut down and stay quiet weakened him to his very bones.

Pulling the bottle of water from his mouth, Max screeched to a halt in the doorway of the sitting room at the same time Carter leaped up from the coach, adjusting his clothing and leaving a very embarrassed Kat in a flustered heap against the cushions. Max remained stock still having no clue what to say or do.

Jesus, wasn't that just the last thing he needed to witness.

"Hey," Carter said quickly, rubbing his hands over his short hair.

"Hey," Max replied, looking between the two guilty faces in front of him.

"Good run?"

Inexplicable yet steady annoyance slinked up Max's throat at Carter's smile and obliviousness. As much as they tried not to shove it in Max's face, happiness exuded from both him and Kat on a sickening scale. And why the fuck shouldn't they be happy? They were getting married; they were in love and content while Max was continuously fighting a horrendous battle against the current of his habit.

He took a deep breath. "Sure."

Without another word, he headed toward the stairs. Dammit, he needed a shower and a stern word with himself. Being pissed because Carter was getting close with his fiancée in his own house was absurd, but shit, there it was. His foundations had been seriously wobbled by his need for a line, and his lack of sleep, making his temper short. He'd made it to his room door when Carter caught up with him.

"I'm sorry, man," he said, making Max turn.

Max rubbed the back of his neck and exhaled, hopelessly trying to rein in his irritation. "No problem," he replied flippantly. "It's your house, right?"

Carter's brow furrowed. "Sure, but it's not fair to— Are you okay?"

Max shrugged petulantly. "As good as every other day when you'd fucking kill for something you can't have." His tone was biting, his words referring to so much more than the coke he yearned for, but, to his credit, Carter didn't react.

"You've spoken with Tate?"

Max bit his tongue, holding back the spiteful retort that bubbled up from the black envy swirling in his belly, and nodded.

"Can I do anything?"

"No." The word was swift and, although Max despised himself for it, laced with bitterness.

The two men stood in silence for a beat before Carter took a step closer. "Look, is now a good time? I have something to ask you. Something important."

The small quiver in Carter's voice had Max on point immediately. "What's wrong?"

"Oh, nothing. No, shit's good, I mean, okay, it's just—you caught us celebrating a little." The way Carter filtered drove Max to distraction. "Kat and I have decided to have the wedding later this year. Here. On the beach."

Max licked his lips and leaned his shoulder against the doorjamb, joy and anger battling through him, exacerbated by the crushing need to sleep for ten days straight and then call his dealer.

"And I want you to be my best man."

Max shouldn't have been surprised by the request. Hell, when he'd proposed to Lizzie, he'd asked Carter the exact same thing. His face had been a fucking picture. The memory gripped Max like a vise, squeezing and taunting, and hitching his breath, throwing him headfirst into the terrors that had taunted him all night. What the hell was going on with him? His mind whirred and his blood sang out for a taste of white fire.

"Would you?" Carter hedged. "What do you think?" His nervousness was entirely uncharacteristic and should have been like a smack upside the head to Max. Instead, it riled him. He had the sudden and ridiculous urge to cry and throw up all at once.

"I, um . . ." Max pressed his fingertips into his eye sockets, desperate to ease the pressure building at the front of his head. "It's just— I'm feeling . . . Carter, I can't . . ."

"Max?"

Carter's voice sounded far away and, just as Elliot's had been in his office that day, as if Max were underwater. A strong hand gripped Max's shoulder, while words he couldn't decipher pummeled his ringing ears. He tried like hell to breathe, relieved that his ass had found something to sit on before he passed out at Carter's feet.

And wouldn't that just be freakin' awesome?

Vaguely aware that Carter was at his side, Max put his head between his knees and asked Carter to grab one of his clonazepam. A pill and a glass of water were thrust under Max's nose before he swallowed it down and lay back, throwing his forearm over his face, and begging for the drug to work its magic fast.

·   ·   ·   ·

Max awoke with a start. On his elbows, halfway under the blankets of his bed, he looked down at himself, still in his running gear, the low light in the room suggesting it was late afternoon. Just as it had been when he'd had a panic attack with Elliot, the headache left over was fierce. On unsteady legs, he reached for a Tylenol and knocked it back dry.

That shit had come out of nowhere. First his terrors, then the craving, then the attack. What was he doing wrong?

He glanced at himself in the bathroom mirror as he threw water onto his face. He looked beat, worn, and so much older than his twenty-eight years. His brown eyes were sunken in their sockets, he hadn't shaved in three days, and his dark hair was a fucking catastrophe of epic unruly proportions. The outside, however, was not a patch on how he felt on the inside. But what the hell else could he do? He'd been taking his meds like a good Boy Scout, exercising, and doing enough to keep his brain from turning to gray mush, but still he'd lost it. Frustration and exhaustion flittered over his skin.

Grabbing his cell phone and firing off a text to Tate asking if he could call and maybe meet up, Max slowly made his way down the stairs, enticed by the delicious smell of chili. Voices floated from the kitchen, hushed and concerned. It wasn't until he was in the doorway of the kitchen, hearing a cell phone chirp with an incoming text, that he realized Tate was sitting at Carter's breakfast bar.

"Hey, you're up," Kat said with a cautious smile from her place by the oven.

Tate's and Carter's heads both snapped toward him. Max fidgeted under their scrutiny. "Yeah. Sorry. Shit got a bit hairy there for a moment." He cleared his throat in embarrassment. He frowned at his sponsor. "What are you doing here?"

Tate lifted from his seat, pulling his cane from where it rested against his stool. "After our talk this morning, I thought I should come and see you. You sounded . . . off. Then Carter called me."

"I was worried," Carter blurted in explanation, compelling Kat to move closer to his side. "I didn't know what to do." She clutched Carter's hand.

Max sighed, guilt teasing his temples. "It's okay. Thank you."

"Look," Kat said to Carter, interrupting the awkward silence that filled the room. "Why don't you and I go and pick up some bread for dinner and leave these two to talk?"

Carter's troubled gaze stayed on Max, but he eventually nodded and made his way out of the kitchen. By the time the front door had closed and the sound of Carter's motorcycle had slowly disappeared into the distance, Max was sitting opposite Tate, clutching a glass of milk in one hand and his head in the other.

"Hell of a day, huh?" Tate began, his voice quiet.

Max closed his eyes, listening to the silence of the house, realization cloaking him. "I can't stay here."

Tate smiled sadly when Max looked up. "Not quite working out how you thought."

His statement hit the nail on the damned head. Max had tried so hard to fit back in. He'd tried to carry on, regardless of the weird feelings of dispassion and disconnection that clutched his heart, but it was no good. Seeing Carter and Kat together after the night he'd had, coupled with the cravings that still burned the back of his throat, had tipped him over the edge. He didn't blame them. Jesus, they'd both done all they could to welcome him into their home and make him comfortable. And yet it simply wasn't enough.

"I don't want to go back to my apartment," Max stated. "I don't want to go back to the city just yet." Besides being too busy and loud for him to deal with, the place was filled to the fucking brim with temptation, reeking of bad history and worse habits.

"I'll support you no matter what you decide," Tate said. "You know what you need better than anyone else. But make sure you're making the decision to better yourself, not because you're scared and running away."

Max scoffed. "But I *am* scared," he confessed. "I'm fucking terrified." His voice broke and he growled in exasperation. "I don't want to let anyone down, or upset anyone. I've done too much of both in my life."

"But this is about what's best for you, Max," Tate urged. "Nobody else. If you need to be selfish, be selfish! And believe me, your friends only want what's best for you."

Max fisted his hair. "I don't want them to think I'm not grateful. I am. I just . . . need to be away from all of this for a while." He sniffed. "I thought I'd started to find myself again, but now I feel more lost than when I fucking started. I don't know *where* I belong."

Tate's hand touched Max's arm. "Then go and find out."

10

The bar was as busy as expected for a game night. The banter and cursing had already begun in earnest as the Orioles fell behind by three, with beer and food being ordered in tandem with each pitch. Not that Grace minded. On the contrary, she'd grown to like the atmosphere of Whiskey's, and the fact that many of the regulars had started to warm to her made it even better. They'd been wary for a while but, thankfully, Holly had been integral to Grace's being accepted into the fray. It was laughable, really, but that was bar politics for you.

"Grace, can I have another draft, please?"

"Sure, Earl," she answered with a smile. "You're not watching the game?"

Earl lifted an unimpressed eyebrow. "Not this bunch of idiots," he huffed. "Let me know when the Washington Nationals are playin' and we'll talk."

"No problem," Grace replied with a laugh as she placed Earl's beer in front of him while simultaneously lifting his ten-dollar bill from the bar.

"Hey, pretty lady. How are you?" Grace smiled shyly at Caleb's greeting as he sat himself down next to Earl at the bar and grabbed a handful of peanuts. She pulled a bottle of Heineken from the fridge and handed it to him.

"I'm good. And you?" She was constantly polite with the deputy; after all, he was a paying customer and he was always pleasant and charming enough. Nevertheless, Kai's distaste for him on his last visit had planted a far from innocuous seed of caution in her belly. Despite Grace's need to prove a point and be free in making her own decisions in life, her momma had always taught both her and Kai to listen to their guts. Not that her gut distrusted the deputy, of course, but she was guarded all the same.

Caleb grinned and dipped his head. "I'm just great. The Baileys' place is looking mighty impressive. Shouldn't be long before you're in there, huh?"

Grace's smile widened. It was true. The building was starting to look like a real, honest-to-God house. Floors were finished, as were the stairs, porch, and walls. Next week was all about the windows and Grace could barely contain her excitement.

"I can't tell you how amazed I am at Vince's work," she replied. "His team is incredible and—"

"Did I hear my name?" Vince Masen, owner of Masen Construction and Masen's Boardinghouse, smirked as he strode toward the bar. He was followed through the entrance by a group of six men whom Grace recognized as workers on the house. She'd seen them all before. Except one. "I hope you're sayin' nice things, Mrs. Brooks," he drawled. "We've just finished up a twelve-hour day on your property."

Grace blushed. "It's Ms., or Grace, and of course I was. I was just telling the deputy here that your work and your team's work has been nothing short of extraordinary. I'm more than grateful."

Vincent Masen was a stocky man with a broad chest that spoke of years of labor and a head of salt-and-pepper hair that made him look distinguished. She guessed him to be in his midfifties but, from what she'd seen since his construction company had begun work on the house, he had the tenacity and the energy of a much younger man. He tilted his chin under her compliment and raised the glass of beer Grace paid for in thanks.

The rest of the guys bought a beer each and ordered food, all except the new face, who stayed at the back of the group, tall, silent, and watching Grace with intense brown eyes that were framed with thick lashes. His irises were so dark they appeared endless in their intensity, like two huge Hershey's Kisses filled with untold secrets. The hair on his head was almost black in the dim light of the bar; it was short at the sides, but long and wild on top, with bits that stuck up as though caught by surprise. His face was hard around the edges and shadowed with stubble that looked a few days old. From the lines around his eyes and mouth, he was either a lot older than Grace imagined, or he'd had a tough life. Either way, his face was not entirely displeasing to look at. Rather like a disheveled Colin Farrell, Grace mused.

Grace tried to smile at him, but he looked away quickly, thanking Vince for the orange juice he handed to him. They made their way across the bar, parked it near the pool table, and set about talking. His shoulders rounded as he sat on his stool, as though trying to make himself smaller while the men around him laughed and chatted.

"Somethin' caught your eye there, honey?"

Holly's voice startled Grace. She was immediately horrified to realize she'd been staring. "No, um, not really. I was just wondering who the new guy was on Vince's team. I haven't seen him at the house."

Holly looked across the bar, narrowing her blue eyes as though it would help her identify the newbie quicker. She shrugged and continued placing the glasses on the correct shelves. "No idea. But it's about time we had something new, male, and pretty to look at around here. Am I right?"

Grace giggled into her hand. The newcomer was certainly easy on the eyes, which undoubtedly surprised her. It had been a long time since she'd felt any flutter of attraction toward the opposite sex, due to the hurt that her past flirtations and intimacies had brought her. Her track record with making sound decisions where men were concerned was not stellar, and with everything that had happened in the past two years, her fear was always enough to help her politely steer clear of any man who showed her even an ounce of attention. Not that this guy had; he hadn't even smiled back.

Caleb turned back to face the bar with a furrow in his brow. "That's Vince's nephew," he added to the conversation. "Didn't catch his name. Flew in from New York a few days ago. He's staying at the boardinghouse here in Preston County." Caleb was silent a beat. "I'd keep a distance, ladies. From what I hear he's had problems, been in prison, involved in some pretty bad shit up there. Drugs and the like. Apparently, he's here to 'clean up.'"

The deputy used his fingers as he spoke to punctuate his meaning and Grace's heart skipped in her chest.

Well, of course, the newbie had a dubious past. What other douches was she attracted to other than those who'd been paroled at least once in their lives and/or were involved in illegal substances? Jesus, she was a magnet for that type of crap. It followed her everywhere. Dammit. She silently cursed her gut, which was evidently not working on all cylinders.

"Okay, then." She huffed out a humorless breath of laughter and picked up a towel to wipe down the bar, counting down the last few hours of her shift and keeping her curious gaze away from Vince's pretty nephew and his intriguing eyes.

• • • •

Max's decision to leave Carter's beach house and fly to Preston County, West Virginia, was, after almost a week, turning out to be a good one. And thank fuck for that. He could already feel the tight ropes of anxiety loosening as he ran through the dense forests behind his uncle's boardinghouse, and not seeing the faces of his past every day eased the tension he'd been carrying like a bag of bricks. Although he felt immeasurably guilty for leaving, his ability to breathe a little easier made it worthwhile.

Just as Tate had predicted, Carter and Kat were both eager for him to do what was necessary to get better, and if that meant he had to leave and stay with his uncle Vince for a while, then so be it. The panic attack that the two of them had witnessed had undoubtedly revealed how far from recovery Max actually was. After Tate had researched and organized a nearby NA meeting for Max to attend, as well as having him placed back on Elliot's list of regular patients at his office in Pittsburgh, Max was set to go within a couple of days. He immediately started to feel better, less stressed, more at ease in his own skin.

His feet pounded the forest floor, his knees and legs burning, while the smell of freshly fallen rain filled his lungs like precious elixir. Following the path down toward the main road, Max slowed and jogged into town, back toward the boardinghouse. Uncle Vince had been more than a little surprised by the phone call Max had made to ask if he could visit. They'd not seen each other for almost eight years—not since Max's father's funeral—but Max knew he'd be welcomed with open arms. Despite Vince not being a relation by blood, he and Max's father had grown up together, always treating each other and their families as true brothers would.

"Maximus Asshat!"

Max came to an abrupt stop at the familiar nickname. He turned to his left where the shout had come from, staring across the street to see his cousin Ruby standing outside her auto body shop, arms open wide.

"Ruby Tuesday!" He flew at her like a bullet, making her squeak in surprise, and grabbed her before she could make a run for it, squeezing her tightly.

"Dad said you were in town," she said with a laugh, hugging him back. "How the hell are you?"

"I'm good," he replied, putting her back down on the ground. "How're you? What the fuck's this I hear about you getting married? I met your hubby when I went to work with your dad yesterday."

She blushed crimson, pushing a hand through her cropped brown hair, and nodded. "Three months." She held out her left hand, the diamond on her third finger small but elegant. "Josh and I sent you an invitation, but . . . I guess you weren't home."

The smile on Max's face dropped minutely. He sighed, knowing that all the dirty details of the past eight years he'd shared with his uncle the day he'd arrived would have been passed on to Ruby within hours. Not that he minded. He'd prefer his family knew the shit he'd done. Nevertheless, small towns were funny places, and variations of his dirty laundry had no doubt been aired several times since his appearance. "Yeah," he replied. "I was . . . unavailable. Sorry."

Ruby placed a hand on his chest and lowered her voice. "But you're getting better?"

"Slowly but surely." Max smiled tentatively.

Ruby's gray eyes softened. "I'm glad." They hugged again, only breaking apart when one of Ruby's workers whistled loudly.

"There she is," a dude with shoulder-length blond hair and tattooed knuckles exclaimed as he stared across the street. "My little RiRi."

Max turned in curiosity to see the same girl who worked behind the bar his uncle had taken him and his other workers to the previous night. She scurried down the street, white earbuds in her ears, a large bag slung over her shoulder, wearing black jeans and a yellow sweater that complemented her dark skin. Her black hair was back in a ponytail that swung from side to side as she walked.

"RiRi?" Max asked with a cocked eyebrow, his stare following the object of Blond Guy's blatant affections.

"Yeah," the man replied with a lascivious lick of his lips. "Her name's Grace, but she looks just like Rihanna, right?"

"No, Buck," Ruby interjected with an eye roll. "She doesn't." She pursed her lips thoughtfully. "She's softer somehow, less sex and more warm hugs." She pushed Buck's arm. "Now quit your hollerin' and get back to work. You'll scare the poor girl to death."

"Oh, man, you wanna see her up close," Buck continued, looking at Max. "Green eyes, mocha skin. Damn fine ass." He wandered back toward an '89 Buick, shaking his head.

Max wasn't knowledgeable enough to comment on the ass thing, not having seen it clearly, but he understood the remark about Grace's eyes. She'd looked at him over the bar last night, the green of her eyes bright and stunning. He'd been momentarily hypnotized by her when they'd entered Whiskey's, and was only shunted from his trance when she'd smiled.

It was, for sure, a very pretty smile, but Max couldn't allow himself to ponder on that too much. He was there to clear his head, not become even more muddled by a strange girl who'd sent an alluring look his way. Of course, he'd be more than happy to satisfy his male urges by fucking her into oblivion if she asked, but just from looking at her for the brief time he had, he knew she wasn't that type of girl. Ruby was right. There was a softness about her. There was too much innocence in those eyes, and maybe a hint of fear, which he was glad of, if it meant she kept her distance.

Max turned back to Ruby, pushing any thoughts of sex or green eyes from his mind. "So are we gonna hang out while I'm here?" he asked.

"Absolutely. I can make dinner. You can meet Josh properly."

Max pulled affectionately on a piece of her hair. "Sounds good."

11

Max's uncle, Vince, opened Masen's Boardinghouse long before Max was born, with his first wife. For the ten years before they divorced they welcomed visitors to the town with good food, hospitality, and a decent bed. Vince's second wife, Fern, Ruby's mom, took on the running of the boardinghouse with little fuss and an expert business eye, while Vince set up what would become Masen Construction. The Masen family had long been an unquestionable force and brought more money into the town than anyone else. To say that Uncle Vince was a hero to the community would have been an understatement.

With a towel around his hips and steam billowing out of the bathroom door behind him, Max wandered back into his room, glancing at the wall-mounted clock to see that it was a little after seven in the morning. He lifted his underwear and jeans from the bed and pulled them on. The room he was staying in was pleasant enough with a large bed, TV, and wardrobes. The floral drapes were not quite to Max's taste, but he'd learn to tolerate them.

He sipped quickly from the cup of coffee he'd made with the standard percolator before pulling on his socks, boots, and a black Sonic Youth T-shirt. He was working for his uncle again— determined to pay for his stay one way or another, even with manual labor, despite his uncle's protestations that Max was there to take it easy and recuperate. But Max had shut down his uncle's concerns. It kept Max's pride from taking a hit with free bed and board, and because his uncle was a stubborn ass and wouldn't take any money, it kept him busy both physically and emotionally, and *that* was always a good thing. His terrors, for the most part, had stayed away, but he wasn't taking any chances.

He sprayed on some deodorant, rubbed the towel over his hair, popped some gum into his mouth, and grabbed his jacket.

Opening the door and vacating the room, he walked smack into something, or rather someone, moving quickly down the hallway. He grabbed at the flailing arms and held whomever it was upright, while cursing under his breath when the toe of their shoe rammed into his shin.

"Oh, God, I'm so sorry!"

Max gained his bearings and looked down at the rushing, apologizing idiot, immediately captured by mesmerizing green eyes and a complete look of surprise. Grace. He released his hold and took a step back. "It's okay. No problem," he muttered, running a hand through his damp hair. Great. Just what he needed first thing in the damn morning.

"I caught your leg," she insisted, a hand at her mouth. "I really am sorry. I wasn't looking where I was going."

"It's fine," he replied, turning from her to lock his door.

"I woke up late because I was working last night and I need to get to the house before the windows arrive. I promised Vince." She continued to ramble even as she reached to the floor to pick up the bag and phone she'd dropped.

Max frowned in confusion. Windows? Vince?

"Are you sure your leg's okay?"

Max exhaled, clutching as much serenity as he could to his chest, and smiled politely. "I've had worse."

Seeming to sense his impatience, she nodded and quickly averted her gaze. "Okay. Well, sorry again." She maneuvered around him, all but darting past like a nervous animal.

Max watched her hurry away, shaking his head wryly when he noticed the ass Buck had mentioned a couple of days before.

Yeah, he was right.

It was slammin'.

Thankfully, Grace was nowhere to be seen when Max finally got outside and to his rental truck. It was an overcast April morning, with the remnants of the night's rainfall gathered in large puddles on the ground. Starting the truck, Max headed away from town toward the site his uncle was working. The project was a huge house, potentially beautiful, set back against the green of the forest. It took only ten minutes in the truck and, when Max arrived, work was well under way.

He waved at his uncle, Josh, and the other guys as he clambered out of the truck and jogged over to where they were unloading a shitload of windows.

"Did ya bring breakfast?" Vince inquired as he heaved a large window from the truck with the help of two other workers.

Max smirked. "'Fraid not."

Vince huffed. "The hell am I payin' you for?"

Max chuckled and got down to work, lugging the windows, timber, and tools up to the house before starting to help with the slow but steady construction of the first-level floors and walls. Hours passed swiftly being so busy. Max's muscles burned gloriously from all the heavy lifting, and the banter with the crew was light. They almost certainly knew who Max was and why he was there, but he couldn't have given less of a shit. They seemed to accept him readily into their team, being Vince's nephew and all, and that, for Max, was enough.

Sitting down in the truck bed opening up his sandwich for lunch with another worker, Rob, Max startled when he noticed Grace speaking with Vince. She was smiling widely, obviously complimenting his uncle on the build work. Max noticed how minute she looked next to Vince's bulky frame and how, bizarrely, she carried an expensive-looking camera around her neck. Maybe she was doing some promo or shit for Vince's company.

Her laugh echoed from where she stood, garnering amorous looks and less than respectful mutterings from others of the work crew. Not that Max blamed them. She looked hot in her yoga pants, sneakers, and sweater. He chuckled when he heard Rob's playful murmurings: "I'm a married man. I'm a married man."

Max pulled his gaze away from Grace, focusing on his bag of chips.

"Y'all okay over here?" Vince asked as he sauntered over and hopped up onto the edge of the truck bed, pulling out his own gargantuan sandwich. Max nodded and smiled around the lip of his bottle of Dr Pepper. "Heard you went to dinner with Ruby and Josh last night."

Max swallowed his drink. "Yeah, it was great seeing her. Plus she made biscuits so I couldn't refuse." Vince laughed. "Josh seems like a nice guy."

"That he is," Vince agreed. "Treats my baby girl right."

"It's a damned good job." Max's eyes once again found Grace, who was taking pictures of the exterior of the house and the sur-rounding forest. He tilted his chin in her direction. "What's she doin' here? She working for you or something?"

Vince scowled in confusion. "No. This is her place. Bought it before Christmas."

Well, shit.

"Don't know much about her," he continued around his balo-ney sandwich. "She's nice and all but keeps herself to herself. I don't know much about her story other than she's paying for all this up front. Must come from money." Vince side-eyed Max and leaned in close. "She's a missus, too, ya know?" He paused for effect. "But there ain't no mister staying with her at the boardinghouse. I'm thinkin' a huge alimony payout."

Max snorted. "You know what they say about gossip, Uncle Vince."

Vince laughed heartily and clapped Max on the back. He gradually quieted and nudged him with his elbow gently. "We haven't had a chance to talk properly, Max. How ya doin'? You feelin' okay bein' here?"

"Yes." The word was out without thought. "I'm okay. I feel . . . better. Less stressed." And it was the truth. "Thank you." Although still restless, he was sleeping better, and his appetite was coming back. He hadn't painted yet, but that would come. "I'm at my NA meeting tomorrow morning. I'll try and get back so I can help out—"

"Max," Vince chastised. "Not that I don't appreciate your thought, son, but it's all right. You come and help me out when you can. You don't have to punch a time clock." He shrugged. "You do what you need to do. Get better. That's what's important right now. That's why you're here."

"I know. I will, but I want to pay my way and—"

"Look," Vince interrupted, turning to look at Max directly, "when he was sick, and even before then when he lost your momma, I promised your daddy that I'd help you whenever I could, or whenever you'd let me. I told him I'd be there just as he promised he'd be there for my Ruby should anything happen to me. Now, I know, like him, you can be a stubborn son of a gun when you want to be." He smiled fondly. "Especially when it comes to accepting help. So imagine how surprised I was when you called."

"Yeah."

"But call you did because somewhere deep inside you knew that, no matter what, I'd be there for you. We all would." He nudged him again. "So let me do this, okay? Let me help."

Max exhaled through a thick throat.

"The only job for you now is to make your daddy proud and get yourself healthy. You hear me, son?"

"Yes, sir." His words were soft and laced with gratitude.

"All right." Vince scrunched up his sandwich packaging and

leaped from the truck bed. "Now, stop sittin' around, eyin' up my clients, and get your ass back to work."

. . .

The NA meeting the following morning was just as Max expected. He sat in the church hall, surrounded by strangers brought together by their dependencies and addictions. He introduced himself, then listened to the unfamiliar faces relay their tales of misery, regret, and recovery. Since his stay in rehab, Max had become a lot more sympathetic to hearing others' stories, so he listened and he understood.

Over the months of his rehabilitation, he'd come to recognize why he'd initially been so closed off from lending an empathetic ear in group. The fact was, every account he heard, every anecdote about hurting loved ones in order to score, and no matter what the consequence, hit close to home. Whether he wanted to or not, Max saw himself in every face of his fellow addicts, the remorse, the cravings that would never ever go away, the need for forgiveness, and the fear of what that forgiveness would mean. He'd never wanted to be *that* guy, the guy who fucked over the people closest to him, the guy who wallowed in self-pity and the what-ifs, but there it was.

He grabbed a cheeseburger for lunch on his contemplative return drive, went for a midafternoon run, and had been in his room at the boardinghouse for more than an hour when a thunderous bang, a squeal of pipes in the wall and the floor, and a scream emitted from the next room.

Max shot from his place on the bed, dropping the book he'd been reading, and flung open the door, scanning the empty hallway. He hurried to the next room, knocking hard, hearing what sounded like water hissing from somewhere and muffled expletives. The door opened abruptly, revealing Grace in nothing but a towel, drenched and breathing heavily.

"The pipe burst!" she exclaimed, leaving the door open for Max to follow, bewildered. "I can't stop it!"

Max hurried into the bathroom after her, his socked feet sloshing in the water that had already gathered. Water spurted forcefully from one of the shower pipes, jetting across the bathroom. "Holy shit."

"Yeah, I agree," Grace said with a laugh. "Help!"

"Go find Fern, um, Mrs. Masen, and tell her to turn off the water and the electric," Max ordered as he motored back to his room. He grabbed his tool belt, willing to try to ease the damage as much as he could, and with a wrench tried to tighten the joint on the pipe.

Water rushed at him, soaking his T-shirt and jeans until, after what felt like a million fucking years, the water stopped, followed by the lights in the bathroom, leaving the place bathed in the dim afternoon light, which crept through a small frosted window. Max slumped against the tub, water dripping from his chin. He cursed, looking down at his sopping wet clothes.

"What in the blue fuck?" Uncle Vince filled the doorway, eyes wide, a small grin tugging at his mouth, as he looked Max over.

Grace popped her head around Vince's shoulder, unable to hold back the unladylike snort that erupted. "Oh, heavens."

"What the hell, Max?" Ruby exclaimed with a giggle. Small chuckles of laughter quickly developed into loud guffaws.

Max shook his head and stood up, careful not to slip. He wiped a dripping hand down his face. "I'm glad I amuse you all."

"That you do. But don't feel bad about it," Vince offered with a hearty slap to Max's shoulder. "Come on. Get changed and let me buy you an orange juice."

•   •   •

Dressed in a dry set of clothes, Max, his uncle, his aunt Fern, Ruby, and Josh sat at the bar in Whiskey's drinking and nibbling potato chips. With the pipe fixed and Grace moved to the room adjacent to Max's while repairs were made to the bathroom floor and bed-room carpet, Max started to see the funny side.

"Hero of the day!" Ruby teased him with an elbow in his ribs, which he returned.

He shrugged, avoiding looking at Grace, who was working diligently behind the bar. She'd done nothing but thank him pro-fusely.

"I always like to save the damsel in distress," he quipped. It'd been on the tip of his tongue to thank Grace for the image of her wet and towel-wrapped, but he managed to refrain.

But, damn, that picture was sure to stay with him a long while; girl had great legs.

"Well, at least I know where you are in case anything else goes wrong," Grace remarked as she wiped down the bar.

"Hey!" Vince interjected with mock offense and a pointed finger at her. "It was a one-time thing. I knew those damn pipes were— Look, nothing else will happen." Aunt Fern rubbed his back, laughing.

"You know where I am," Max stage-whispered across the bar to Grace, who giggled into the back of her hand.

And the banter continued. Max clutched his glass of juice, threw the occasional chip or peanut into his mouth, nibbled on the few wings Vince ordered, and allowed the warmth of the people around him to seep into his skin. It had been too long since he'd felt as relaxed. With his meeting and the exciting burst-pipe shenanigans, he'd been wound tight as shit, but the smiles, laugh-ter, and freedom he felt as he listened to his family and the other patrons loosened all of that. Even being in a bar with the smell of liquor, undeniably tempting around him, Max felt his body unfurl and calm.

"Sounds like a lot of fun was bein' had over at your place, Vince." A tall guy with a goatee and a distrustful gaze patted Vince's shoulder, his eyes never leaving Max.

Vince laughed and relayed the day's events, garnering another round of laughter.

"So *you're* Max," Goatee said with an outstretched hand. "Deputy Sheriff Caleb Yates."

Ah.

Well, that explained the stink-eye.

Max shook his hand, smirking at the slight squeeze the deputy gave it.

"I've known Caleb here since he was in junior high; his daddy worked for me for many years," Vince offered. "Never thought I'd see this guy all but running the town, though."

The deputy chuckled. "Can I get a Heineken draft, Grace?" he muttered over the bar. He winked at her when she placed it down in front of him. "You look sweet tonight." Max watched Grace's reaction carefully from the corner of his eye, but saw no blush or flutter of lashes. If anything she appeared to tense up, losing the softness of her pretty face.

"Flattery will get you nowhere, Deputy. You know that. You still need to pay me a tip," she remarked, making Max smile into his glass.

"Are you okay with that?" she asked suddenly, gesturing to Max's almost empty glass. "I could buy you a beer to say thank you for today." She looked toward the ceiling, her nose scrunching endearingly. "And to apologize for the other day."

Max shook his head, smiling. "No beer. But another juice would be good. Thanks."

"The other day?" Fern asked, looking between them. "What the hell else trouble are you two getting into?"

Grace chuckled. "It was all my fault. Again. Damn near knocked Max over on his ass; I was hurrying down the hallway so fast. Gave his shin a good kick, too, while he held me up."

Despite the laughter and comments, Max could feel the deputy's stare burning into the side of his face. His expression was amused, though his eyes were dark and suspicious.

"Held her up, huh?" he asked, leaning his elbow on the bar.

Max cocked an eyebrow. Asshole was as transparent as the glass in his hand. "Yeah," he answered.

Deputy Yates nodded slowly, glancing at Grace. "Sounds like you're Grace's hero of the hour."

Grace's face flushed. "Oh, no. It wasn't like that, I—"

"Sounds like it," Max interrupted, keen to make the deputy squirm. And squirm he did. A muscle in his jaw jumped and a huff of breath shot from his nose. The deputy swigged from his beer once, dropped a ten on the bar, said his good-byes, and left.

Max couldn't explain it, but watching the deputy leave so affronted, and seeing the small smile on Grace's face, left a more than satisfied taste in his mouth.

12

Max O'Hare was an enigma.

Since she'd fallen into him and he'd then saved her from the demon pipe burst, Grace had thought regularly about him. As the weeks passed, and in spite of the deputy's warning about Max's less than golden past, Grace allowed herself to approach him with tentative familiarity. She spoke to him when he sat at the bar and now knew that his go-to drink was OJ, and greeted him when she encountered him in the boardinghouse or at the house site.

He wasn't as aloof or evasive as he'd been when she'd first come across him, but his guard was still unquestionably up. Bizarrely, instead of seeing his distance as a reason to step back, Grace found herself even more intrigued. With forced indifference and the occasional smile to the bar regulars and even Max's aunt Fern, Grace had discovered that Max had been to rehab for more than three months. She didn't know what for—though Deputy Yates had mentioned drugs—and, the more she thought about it, the more she realized it was irrelevant.

Surely what was important was that he'd gotten help and wanted to be healthy. At least that's what Grace told herself when searching to explain her continuing interest in him.

The thing was, when Max was with his family, or when he thought no one was looking, his barriers dropped. It was only ever for the briefest of moments but when they did they revealed a more contented, less edgy guy who, there was no denying, had a killer smile. Grace knew without a doubt that he'd look great on film. She'd spent time considering the photographs she could take of him.

He was never eager to be the center of attention. Even over Easter, when the boardinghouse had been filled with people, food, and laughter, he'd be sitting on the periphery watching and listening to everyone else, which Grace found . . . attractive. There was nothing worse than an attention-seeking idiot who loved the sound of his own voice. He was quiet, but not brooding, rather the epitome of the strong and silent type.

And unlike the deputy and others who came into the bar, Max was never flirty. He never made unsubtle comments about the way she looked or called her anything other than her name. On occasion, Grace had caught him looking at her in that sideways, inconspicuous way of his and every time it made her stomach twist. Yet he maintained his distance.

Grace wasn't ignorant to her looks. She knew she was attractive to members of the opposite sex. It had been a privilege, before her ex-husband walked into her life and made her believe that being beautiful was something to be ashamed of. Nevertheless, men still stared, smiled, and sometimes commented, but not Max. He remained resolutely apathetic. He was polite, and pleasant, but never showed an interest, and Grace fought to understand why that bothered her so damned much.

She sighed and sipped from her glass of water after telling her therapist as much.

Despite moving to Preston County, West Virginia, the birthplace of her mother, Grace continued her therapy appointments every other week, commuting back to DC by bus and train. She'd stay at Kai's apartment and travel back the following morning. Her brother was clearly not happy about the arrangement—worrying endlessly about her being on her own—but Grace enjoyed the time the journey gave her. Sometimes she read, listened to music, sometimes she took discreet photographs out of the window or of other, more interesting-looking passengers; other times she used it as a chance to reflect on the last few years of her life, especially the changes and the huge strides she'd made in her recuperation.

Two years ago, the thought of traveling alone, never mind by public transport, would have caused a crippling panic attack. Now, as long as she took her meds ahead of time, she didn't even suffer palpitations. It was freeing in a way she could never describe.

"Let me ask you," her therapist, Nina, said gently. "What do you want to achieve from this interest in Max? What is your goal?"

Grace frowned. "My goal?"

"I mean, is this a lust thing, a companionship thing? Do you want to sleep with him or do you just want be his friend?"

Grace shifted embarrassedly in her seat. "He's good-looking, yes, but—sleep with him?" She watched in alarm as the goose bumps popped up on her arms, as they were prone to do at the mere mention of sex. "I can't answer that."

"Is that due to your latent apprehensions toward intimacy or about Max himself?"

Grace wasn't sure. His fleeting glances notwithstanding, she didn't even know if Max was attracted to her. Besides, he'd been through his own rough times and was, according to rumor, staying with his uncle to help his recovery; sex was probably the last thing on his mind.

"I'd like to be his friend," she answered eventually. "With everything he's been through, he might need another one. I know I do."

Nina lifted her chin, watching Grace in that all-knowing way of hers. "Grace, this is the first time since we started these sessions twenty-eight months ago that you've mentioned a man other than your brother or your ex-husband, and what's even more encouraging is that you're attracted to him. Regardless of where you decide to take this, or whether he wants the same thing, remember, this is a step in the right direction."

That Grace had to agree with. Whether it was the house project or the West Virginia air that had bolstered her confidence, she was gradually coming to realize that she no longer wanted to shy away from the prospect of a connection with someone. What that connection might be, she wasn't entirely certain, but for the first time in too long, the unknown was suddenly very exciting.

· · · ·

It was two days after her therapy session before Grace saw Max again. Seated in the window of the coffee shop in town, he sat by himself, pencil in hand with a small sketchbook. His hair fell forward, hiding his eyes while he wrote or drew or whatever the hell he was doing. With her daily latte in one hand and a chocolate muffin in the other, Grace approached, coughing gently so as not to surprise him. He looked up, uncertainty covering his face.

His eyes were darker than usual, circled with tired, bluish bruise-like lines, as though he hadn't slept in a week.

"Hey," she said brightly. "How are you?" There was no answer but for the confused furrow in the center of his brow. She pushed on regardless. "I love the lattes here. Sure beats the hell out of the crap you get in DC."

He glanced at her cup, then at his own, seemingly waking from whatever daze she'd disturbed him in. Grace held her breath.

"I miss the coffee in New York," he murmured.

Success!

"I can imagine," she offered, pressing her lips together. "New York does great coffee. And bagels. Awesome bagels. So . . . may I join you?" She gestured to his book still lying open on the table; she was unable to clearly make out the scribbles and doodles on the pages. "I don't want to disturb or intrude if you'd rather be on your own."

Max closed the book quickly and pulled it toward his body protectively. Slowly, he nodded. "No, it's okay."

He pushed the pencil behind his ear as she sat, and folded his large arms over his broad chest. His size should have been intimidating and Grace didn't doubt that to many it would be, but, oddly, to her, it wasn't. She'd seen him at the site, saw how he used his strength to do his work quickly and effectively, but also saw how, in social situations, he was the complete antithesis, forever trying to make himself look smaller, as though trying to hide or melt into the walls around him. She wondered what had happened in his past that would make him feel it necessary to do that.

"Wanna share?" She pushed the muffin to the center of the table. Max cocked an eyebrow. "Come on," Grace said with a chuckle. "They're really good. I have one every morning." He regarded the muffin questioningly. "I haven't got cooties," she assured him, breaking off a piece and throwing it into her mouth.

Max smiled wryly and, after a moment, did the same. "Thanks."

Grace grinned. "Sure. I haven't seen you for a couple of days. I'd started to panic about what I'd do if the pipes in my new room burst." He snorted. "You must be busy." She stirred her drink after pouring in some more sugar. Her monthly need for all things sweet was kicking her ass.

Max shrugged. "Not really. My uncle said he didn't need me at the house—your house, so I've been . . . hanging out." He stared at the table. It was hard for Grace not to see the sadness, which draped his shoulders like a heavy blanket.

"Hanging out is good," she replied, smiling. "It must be so nice being here with family. They all seem great."

"They are."

"Do you visit them often?"

"No." He glanced out the window; the sun streaming through it made his dark hair lighter, highlighting flecks of gold. "It's been a while. Do you have family here?"

Surprised by the question, but encouraged by his engagement

with the conversation, Grace beamed. "My momma was from West Virginia, that's why I came back here, but we grew up in California, where my daddy came from. Since they died it's just me and my brother, who lives in DC."

Max's face creased with apology.

"It's okay," she assured him. "I miss them both, but life moves on, right?"

His eyes widened, while the right side of his mouth twitched with the beginnings of that glorious smile Grace liked so much but rarely saw. He stole another piece of muffin. "That it does." He lifted his drink, displaying a smudge of black paint on the elbow of his gray Henley.

Grace pointed to it. "You paint?"

His intense gaze snapped to hers, pinning her to her chair. She waved toward the stain and watched as he inspected it. He exhaled, appearing uncomfortable with her discovery and, with the edge of his thumb, began scratching at it in an effort to remove it. "Yeah, I dabble."

"I'd love to see some of your work." Before he could object, she continued. "I was never a painter. That was always Momma. Kai, my brother, he draws, but I was always the one with a camera." Max remained silent, but his stare never wavered. He listened intently, as he always did when she chattered to him over the bar at Whiskey's. "I went to college and studied photography, set up my own business, but then—well, I kinda quit, but I still take my camera everywhere I go." She opened her bag and showed him the Nikon sitting in its depths.

"I saw you taking pictures at the house. Why did you quit?"

The million-dollar question. Grace's shoulders pinched and her finger circled the lip of her cup as she tried to stop her mind from wandering down that particularly horrendous road of her past. As much as she wanted to get to know Max, she wasn't ready to tell him that part of her story. "Life happened."

The answer, as vague as it was, appeared to appease Max's curiosity. "Yeah, it has a way of doing that."

"Sure does," she agreed. "Just jumps up out of nowhere and takes the feet from under you and you lie there wondering what the hell just happened." Even though she tried to keep her voice upbeat, Grace watched as something wretched and broken flashed across Max's face, before the barrier he carried around with him snapped shut behind his eyes, darkness clouding him once again.

Damn. Chitchat over.

He cleared his throat and picked up his book. "I've got to be someplace," he muttered, standing from his seat. "It was nice to see you. Thanks for the muffin."

Grace smiled at his politeness, even with the disappointment that bloomed in her chest. "Oh, yeah, sure." He wasn't always so flustered, fidgety. If anything, it was Max's stillness that she found so entirely fascinating. Something was different.

She watched him retreat quickly out of the coffee shop, his strong shoulders tense, rounded, and his long legs striding purposefully across the street toward his truck. He pushed a hand through his messy hair, once, twice, before climbing into the vehicle and peeling away.

• • • •

Seven hours later, Grace was more than surprised when Max wandered into Whiskey's with two guys she recognized from the work site. He dipped his chin in her direction and parked himself on a stool by the bar while his friends strolled over to the pool table.

"Orange juice?" she asked, trying not to notice his shadowed expression. Whatever had been bothering him at the coffee shop had apparently not been rectified and now shrouded him with a dangerous quiet. He looked ready for a fight.

"No. A shot of Jack," he said, slapping a twenty onto the bar.

Bourbon? This was new. And potentially catastrophic. Grace

had no idea whether Max was a recovering alcoholic or what the hell he was, and a shot of Jack would be a colossal leap off the proverbial wagon. She didn't want to be responsible for that. Grace quickly scanned the bar for Vince, but he wasn't there. Neither was Holly, who she was filling in for, for another two hours. Apart from Max's friends and two other groups of regulars, the place was quiet.

She tapped her fingers on the bar top. "You sure?"

Max's eyes narrowed. "Yeah. Why?"

Grace nibbled her bottom lip. "I just . . . should you be drinking?" Jesus, how awkward could it get? "With you—I mean, you always drink juice."

Understanding flittered over Max's face and a bark of humorless laughter erupted from his chest. His stare was unfriendly and angry and nothing like what she'd faced in the coffee shop. "I'm not a drunk, Grace," he spat. "I'm a fucking drug addict."

"Oh." Grace swallowed that piece of information as though it were a razor blade.

She knew too well the damage drugs could do. She also knew Max really shouldn't be drinking. Substituting one addiction for another was something she knew plenty about.

"So," Max continued with a sarcastic wave toward the bottles of spirits. "Unless the bourbon around here is laced with narcotics, which, I'll be honest, would be fucking stupendous, I'd like a shot of it, if it's all the same to you."

His words weren't mean, but the tone he used was. It skittered down Grace's spine and left her cold. It wasn't as though she and Max were friends, as much as she wanted them to be, but the man sitting in front of her wasn't who she'd grown to know. He was volatile, and sharp, and unsettled Grace to her very bones. Without another word, she turned and poured the drink. She placed it on the bar and watched as he took it from her, staring at it as if it were a grenade about to detonate.

Minutes passed and still he stared at the drink. His lips moved in inaudible mutterings until with a loud "fuck it" he knocked the drink back. He hissed, cursed, and coughed, but the slam of the shot glass back on the wood bar was triumphant. "Another," he ordered.

Grace's heart clenched for him and the war blatantly raging within his head. "Max, honey, why—"

"Are you deaf?" he snapped, glaring at her. "Do your job and keep the drinks coming, okay? I don't need a friend or a chat. I need to get shitfaced. That's all."

Wounded by his sharp tongue, Grace poured the drinks and he shot them.

Time and again he sat with the drink between his hands before he'd knock it back and, time and again, Grace's urge to cry for him and the memories his actions evoked inside her intensified. His buddies from the site did nothing to help. They bought several rounds of drinks, as well as inviting a group of three girls over to join them. Although normally so indifferent to the women who approached him in Whiskey's, tonight Max eyed the girls in a way that made Grace nauseous. It was feral and hungry.

Was this the dangerous stranger Deputy Yates had warned her about?

Was *this* the real Max O'Hare?

She didn't know.

All she did know, when she watched Max stagger out of the bar hours later with his arm wrapped around an eager blonde thing with googly eyes and her hands on Max's ass, was that the tiny piece of hope she'd kept deep inside, waiting patiently for someone good enough to share it with, had splintered into a thousand pieces.

13

There was banging.

Loud fucking banging that rattled Max's already hurting brain within his very skull. He lifted his head from his pillow, and damn if it wasn't a lead weight, squinting against the sunlight pouring through the open drapes.

"Max, open the door."

Motherfucker.

Tate.

"Max." His voice was hard, angry. "I don't give a shit if I am a cripple; I *will* break this door down. United States Marine Corps, asshole. Let's go. Get your stupid ass up. I don't care if you're naked, either. I'll shoot whatever the fuck I've not seen before." He hammered the door further. "Now, Max. Get up! I know you're in there."

The room tilted like a freaking roller coaster when Max sat up and his stomach sloshed in a way that really didn't feel good or normal. He stood on wobbly legs, pulled a pair of jeans over his underwear, and stumbled to the door, kicking a pizza box and an empty bottle of Jack out of the way.

"All right," he croaked as he rested his forehead against the door and unlocked it. He took a deep breath and pulled the door open. When he saw Tate's expression, he really wished he hadn't.

"Morning, Starshine," Tate snapped. "What. The. Actual. Fuck?"

Max leaned his cheek against the door's edge, trying to put

into words and full sentences just exactly what he'd been thinking when he went to the bar last night and drank his body weight in liquor.

"Get dressed," Tate said. "We're going out."

Max glanced at his watch. It was past noon but he could easily have slept for another twelve hours. "Tate, man, I can't, I need—"

"No," Tate barked, his eyes flashing with a disappointment that made Max want to go fetal. "I've driven two hours to get here. I'm tired and I need coffee and I don't give a shit about your hangover."

Lacking the energy to argue back, and knowing he was the dickhead Tate was implying he was, Max pulled a clean T-shirt from a drawer, pulled on his boots, grabbed his wallet and his jacket, and headed out of the door, wishing the sledgehammer sticking in the front of his head would just back the fuck off.

Max directed Tate into town, unable to drive them himself, and to the coffee shop he frequented, ordering the strongest coffee on the menu, as well as a chocolate muffin. They sat at the same table he'd been sitting at when Grace had joined him the day before. Max's headache strengthened at the thought of her. Jesus. She must think him an absolute prick. He *was* an absolute prick.

"So you wanna explain to me why I got a phone call from you at two o'clock this morning, at three o'clock this morning, and at four o'clock this morning?" Tate asked, showing him the missed-calls list on his cell phone. "As well as several texts telling me how much you wanted to drink yourself to death, how you couldn't stay clean, how you were giving up?" Tate dropped his cell to the table and crossed his arms over his chest, serious and stern despite the T-shirt he wore, which read "A salt with a deadly weapon" underneath a picture of a salt shaker holding up a gun to a pepper shaker.

Max dropped his forehead to his forearm on the table and groaned. He only had a vague recollection of speaking to Tate. In regard to the texts, he was fucked if he could remember. "Christ, man, I'm sorry," he mumbled before sitting up again. "If it's any consolation, I feel like death wrapped in shit, wrapped in death. I'm really fucking sorry."

"Don't be sorry," Tate retorted firmly. "Tell me what the hell happened."

Vomit crept up Max's throat. He took a huge gulp of coffee to chase it back down. "Yesterday was . . . Lizzie—it was when she left. It was the date of when she left me."

"And instead of calling you decided to deal with that little detail by getting hammered," Tate stated. "Great choice. I see your time in rehab has really helped you make spot-on decisions. You drank your weight in alcohol while on antidepressants and all the other pills that—"

Max's temper flared. "Fuck you, okay, I had a bad day, and I wanted a drink." His curse and loud voice brought the attention of the other patrons to their table. Glancing around quickly, Max swallowed and took a breath. When he spoke again, it was quieter but still angry. "I shouldn't but I did. I know for damn certain I'm not the first it's happened to. You can't sit there all fucking self-righteous, either, when you know you did the same. I can't change it. It is what it is."

"No," Tate argued. "It isn't. Yes, I fucked up when I first left rehab, too. And I'm gonna tell you exactly what my sponsor told me: *You* have the choice, Max. *You* have the tools to make a good decision, to fight against days like yesterday. You have people who care about you, who want what's best for you, and you can't afford to forget that."

Max clasped the bridge of his nose and sighed. He did know it. He knew he'd let everyone down, he knew it was a setback after months of hard work and fight. It was just that some days the fight in him just wasn't enough.

"Open your wallet," Tate said.

Too dizzy and tired to ask why, Max pulled his wallet from

his jeans pocket and handed it to his sponsor. Tate opened it and pulled out the five NA medallions Max had received.

Tate pushed them into a circle. "These show how far you've come," he said, his voice quieter. "These show the choice you made five months ago when you grabbed your addiction by the balls and said 'screw you, bitch, I'm fighting this.'"

Max held his head in his hands. "It's hard sometimes."

Tate scoffed. "No shit. It's hard all the time, Max. All the time. And it'll continue being hard for the rest of your life, because that's what we, as addicts, have to survive. You think I still don't have bad days? Days where I just want to call my old dealer or steal a prescription and get dosed? I do." He stared at the coffee cup between his hands. "But then I remember what that would do to my parents, my family, and my friends. To me. And that's what *you* need to do."

"I did," Max mumbled. "I knew this day was coming. I haven't slept all week. I've had nightmares like you wouldn't believe, even with my meds. I painted for the first time since I got here. I went for a run, I tried to sleep, to read, I called Carter, Elliot, but it was like a fucking lead weight around my neck. I couldn't breathe. The only thing I knew would ease it was a line." He grimaced. "So I went to the bar to find the next-best thing."

The two men sat in silence, both drained by their respective struggles. "Max, I get it," Tate offered quietly. "You know I do. But these days will happen. They'll poleax you and leave you desperate to throw your medallions away. But, I promise you, one day you'll wake up and you won't think about a line, or a pill, or any kind of fucked-up high first. You'll find something that makes you want to leap out of bed in the morning and say 'come on life, bring it, I'm ready.'"

Max picked a chocolate chip off his muffin and put it in his mouth. Grace was right. They were good, even with more alcohol in his veins than actual blood.

"Promise me next time you'll call me before you get to the bar, not when you leave it," Tate urged.

"Next time?"

"There'll be many. That's a fact."

And didn't that sound superfun? Max nodded despondently.

"Good. Now call Elliot for an emergency appointment."

Max gaped. "I can't. It's Sunday."

"Like I give a shit. Besides, I already called him first thing. He's expecting you and he's already on his way. Come on." Tate stood, clutching his cane in one hand and his coffee in the other. "I'll drive."

·   ·   ·

By the time Tate dropped Max back at the boardinghouse, it was early Sunday evening. The session with Elliot had been as hard as Max expected, although being prescribed stronger meds to help him sleep was a bonus. He didn't doubt, however, that with his hangover still teasing the edges of his brain and his stomach filled with Mickey D's, he'd sleep like a fucking baby. Before he dropped fully dressed back into bed, however, Max knew he had to apologize to Grace. He'd spoken to her like a shit and, despite not knowing her all that well, he knew she didn't deserve his temper. No one did.

So, with an uneasy fidget in his shoulders and nerves in his gut, he knocked on the door of her room.

"Just a minute!" Grace called from inside.

Max rubbed his forehead with the back of his hand and waited.

Why the hell was he putting himself through this again?

Oh, yeah.

Because he was an asshole.

Because Elliot had explained how important it was to apologize for his mistakes, so he could move through life without any regrets.

Because the NA Step Working Guide taught addicts how they had to own up to their behaviors.

Because Grace was a nice girl.

The door opened with a flourish to wide green eyes that were immediately suspicious.

"Hey," Max said when she remained silent.

She exhaled hard, her shoulders dropping, her face hardening.

That right there was why he had to say sorry.

"Hey."

Max shifted his weight from foot to foot under her glare, his eyes traveling from the loose ponytail in her hair, to her makeup-free face, and down her body. She was wearing running gear, a pastel pink vest, and tight black running pants that clung to her in ways that should be illegal. She was barefoot, the polish on her dainty toes matching her top.

"I, um, I'm sorry to bother you," he stammered. "I hope you weren't busy, but I wanted to give you these." He held out a takeout coffee cup and a white paper bag.

She eyed them distrustfully, crossing her bare arms over her chest. "And what are these?"

Max shrugged and lifted the cup. "A peace-offering latte"—he lifted the bag—"and an apology muffin."

Grace frowned, still not taking either. "What are you apologizing for?"

He sighed, his arms falling under the weight of his guilt. "I'm apologizing for being a bad-tempered asshole. I shouldn't have spoken to you like that; I put you in a really awkward position and I shouldn't have." He lifted the gifts again, smiling timidly.

She seemed to consider his apology for a freakin' age before she reached out and took them with a small "thanks."

"You're welcome," he replied, pushing his hands into the back pockets of his jeans.

"I'll have them when I get back."

He gestured to her attire with a lift of his chin. "You're going for a run?"

"Yeah," she answered, the usual brightness slowly filtering back into her voice. "I have to fight off the chocolate calories somehow."

"Sure," he replied. "I go running, too. There's a great route down by the stream."

Her expression became animated, her smile wide and beatific. "Maybe you could show me. I like having company when I run and I'm still learning the area."

The sound that came from Max's gullet was not a good one. "I'll have to pass," he murmured, toeing the floor. "I'm not feeling too great."

Grace's smile fell. "Oh, yeah. Well, anyone who can drink that much whiskey is bound to have the mother of all hangovers the day after."

Max cleared his throat of the embarrassment that teased it. "Yeah."

"And your girlfriend, was she feeling crappy this morning, too?"

Max's head snapped up so quick he almost toppled over. Shit. The blonde. Of course, she saw him with her. He'd told the boys he wasn't interested in hooking up with anyone, but they hadn't listened, which was fine because after his seventh and eighth drink an anonymous fuck sounded pretty awesome to him, too.

"I don't— No, I don't . . . she's not, we were just hanging out. Nothing—it wasn't like that."

He had no idea why he was rambling or why he felt the need to explain himself. The truth was, the girl *had* tried to get in his pants, and he'd been quite happy for her to, until she tried to kiss him on the mouth and call him baby. That put the brakes back on his libido right quick. That shit was far too intimate, too close to memories he was working to erase. Besides, it wasn't as if he could get a hard-on anyway, what with the gallons of liquor sloshing through his system.

He'd walked her home, bought a bottle of Jack and a pizza, and headed back to the boardinghouse, where he'd apparently called Tate a million and one times.

"Well, thanks for these," Grace said, avoiding his eyes. "I appreciate the gesture."

She turned to go, but Max caught the door with the palm of his hand, startling her. "Sorry," he blurted. "I was just . . . I'm sure I'll feel better tomorrow. I could show you the route then. If you want. If you're not busy or whatever."

What the hell was it about this woman that had his tongue in a fucking twist? And why the hell was he offering to share his run with her? Unlike her, he loved the solitary quiet of the route he ran every day. Grace would no doubt chatter away like a fucking chattering thing, shattering the serenity he tried so hard to cling to. She'd want to talk and shit and he'd just want to run—what the hell was he thinking?

She blinked at him a couple of times before her lips twitched with another smile. "That sounds nice."

That pulled Max up short, because seeing her normal soft, happy face instead of the disappointed hurt she'd worn when she opened the door was worth losing the quiet of just one run.

"Well, all right," he said with a nod, because, honestly, how bad could it be?

*   *   *

They met the following day in the corridor between their rooms.

Awkwardly, they set off from the boardinghouse, Max leading the way through the back paths, through the forest, and down toward the stream that ran the length of the entire town. His earbuds remained dangling from where they sprouted out of the neck of his T-shirt, bouncing against his chest as he ran. He didn't want to be rude and listen to music, in case Grace wanted to talk, but, to his surprise, she remained at his side or behind him when the path became too narrow, quiet, and focused.

She kept up with him, too. She met him stride for stride and didn't look as ready as Max when they stopped for a water break.

"This place is beautiful," she whispered, taking in the high canopy of green above them. "I've been here for months and never knew all this was so close."

"I love it out here," Max confessed, before chugging his water. It was true. It was so quiet, fresh, and green, especially now that it was the middle of spring.

"I could take some amazing photographs." She let her hand whisper across the moss of a nearby tree.

Before Max could comprehend what she was doing, or ask her more about her photography, she reached into her vest top and pulled out her phone. He stood mesmerized, openmouthed. "You just pull that out of your bra?"

"And it's a sport's bra, lemme tell you, it's far from comfortable. I'll no doubt have the Apple logo creased into the skin of my boob for days." Grace snorted at Max's dumbfounded expression and set about taking pictures of the trees, spiderwebs, and flowers.

"You can take good pictures on that thing?" he asked, scratching his head, trying to rid himself of the image of Grace rustling around in her bra, around her Apple-marked boobs for her phone. Christ, she was something else. It was bad enough watching her run in all that skintight Lycra. And, of course, bad meant good, because, seriously, the woman was wearing that shit like it was her job, all curvy, soft shapes, lean legs, and—

"They're not bad," she answered, leaning over to get a shot of . . . something. "But it's more to give me an idea of color and light. I'll come back with my real camera."

They set off again five minutes later. Their pace was good and they were on their way back to town within the hour. Max slowed to a stop when Grace called out. He turned to see her grabbing her right side and then her hip, flinching.

"You okay?" He jogged back.

She waved him off. "Yeah, yeah. I just . . . I have an old injury that flares up sometimes. It'll pass. Go on, keep going, I know my way back from here."

"It's fine," he assured her. "I've hit my miles. I don't mind walking."

They walked the rest of the way back to the boardinghouse. Max listened to Grace wax lyrical about her job at Whiskey's, how having a job was so important to her, and how excited she was about the house and the progress the workers were making. Max listened, wondering exactly how she found such joy and delight in everything. He'd never met anyone who saw such positivity in everyday things; even his asshole behavior seemed to have been forgiven and forgotten.

Her outlook was refreshing and, Max had to admit, infectious. He found himself smiling as she talked, watching her hands move frantically as she described how she wanted to decorate and furnish her house. He didn't doubt that, without her hands, she'd be rendered mute.

"Maybe I could buy one of *your* paintings," she commented. "A Max special. I could give it pride of place in my living room."

Max rubbed the back of his neck nervously. "Maybe."

"What do you paint about?" she asked, her tone interested as opposed to nosy. She kept her eyes on the path ahead.

"Stuff," he replied petulantly. He noticed the exasperated look she threw him. "I vent," he added. "About things that I went through. When I was . . . in rehab, I attended art therapy sessions. It helped me express what I couldn't in group or with my shrink."

Max surprised himself with the outpouring of information and the fact that he didn't feel vulnerable sharing with Grace. He didn't know her all that well, and to share so freely was new for him. She didn't respond but she didn't look anything other than attentive, which she always did when he spoke.

"It's great that you have that," she said eventually.

They reached the boardinghouse, climbed the stairs to the first level, and stood at their respective doors, once again awkward and fidgety.

"I enjoyed today," Grace said, tapping her finger on her door handle. "Thanks."

"Me, too," Max replied, and, weirdly, it was the truth.

"We'll have to do it again sometime."

"Sure."

"Maybe tomorrow?"

"Why not? Tomorrow."

14

In fact, tomorrow's run turned into a run the day after, and the day after that, and the day after that. Every afternoon of the following two weeks, once Max was finished at the site, or in the morning before Grace went to work at the bar, they ran the same route, through the forest and down by the stream. They ran, Grace photographed some more, and they talked, but never about anything too deep or serious. It was banter and it was fun.

Over the days that followed, Grace learned that Max had lived in New York for most of his life. His best friend was getting married at the end of the summer, and Max was going to be the best man. He loved cars and owned a body shop, played acoustic guitar, loved rock music, and, despite his modesty when it came to his artistic talents, he knew about colors and techniques, better than he let on. She knew he was an orphan, but didn't push on the details and steered clear of anything to do with his rehab, although she knew his therapist's name, and he talked about his sponsor, Tate, frequently.

Since he'd knocked on her door, shocking the hell out of her with his apology and a chocolate muffin, Grace had started to see more of Max O'Hare's sunnier side. With each day that passed, he became less dark, more relaxed, and that smile she liked so much started to come easier. She liked making him laugh, too—the sound forever wrapped around her like a warm hug—and tried to do it as often as she could. He looked so much younger when he laughed, less weighed down by life.

Unlike other men Grace had come across since her ex-husband, Grace didn't feel anxious around Max. On the contrary, in Max's presence she felt calm and safe. She couldn't deny the night he'd been so abrasive at the bar had been horrible, but the more time she spent with him, the more she came to understand how out of character his mood had been. She knew too well how the mood swings of addicts were unpredictable and erratic and, if she and Max were going to be friends, she had to be prepared for that.

Maybe she *was* a lunatic for wanting to know him better, just as Kai had exclaimed on the phone when she'd mentioned Max. Maybe she *was* a glutton for punishment getting involved with a man who was a recovering drug addict, but she couldn't find it in herself to worry or care. The truth was she liked him. He was handsome, funny, and honest.

One particular afternoon, as she took more photographs of her house, which was mere weeks from completion, she caught herself watching him and the way he moved. Unlike when he was running, when his jaw was hard, his dark eyes focused, and his muscled arms and legs propelled him forward with speed and certainty, on the site his broad shoulders were looser, his hips similar. He was graceful, light, and, admittedly, sexy as hell.

He'd dip his chin if she caught his eye, a familiar acknowledgment, which always made Grace smile. He wasn't entirely indifferent to her when they weren't running, he was still unfailingly polite, but he did keep his distance. And Grace liked it. She liked knowing she had access to another side of him when it was just the two of them. She liked that they had something that was theirs and no one else's. It wasn't a secret, but she accepted that, should anyone hear about their meetings every day, they would assume something more was going on. Something dirty and impure, and that would spoil everything.

"That's a pretty smile," Deputy Yates commented from his stool, as she poured him a beer at Whiskey's that evening. "Who's it for?"

Grace shrugged and placed the glass in front of him. "Life's just good right now," she replied. "My house looks amazing; I've made some great new friends."

The deputy nodded and sipped his drink, leaving a small line of white foam in the hair over his top lip. "You seem to like that O'Hare fella a whole lot. I saw you together at the coffee shop last week."

Grace sighed. "Yeah, he's a nice guy," she commented dismissively.

A husky voice floated from the far end of the bar. "I'll say he's a nice guy. Hot as Hades, too. I can't wait for round two with that man."

The blonde woman Max had left Whiskey's with propped herself against the bar, elbows bent, her lips painted a bright red that washed out her skin. She smiled at Grace in a way that was neither nice nor genuine. It was more like a sneer that made Grace's spine straighten. Blondie pushed her boobs together, resting them on her forearms on the bar top, giving the other patrons an eyeful. In her tight vest top and even tighter jeans, she was all hard fucking and dirty passion with no limits. She was everything Grace would never be.

Deputy Yates scoffed. "Jesus, Fay, you don't change. He ain't a nice guy. I don't trust him."

But Grace wasn't listening.

She was too busy trying to delete the vision of Max and Fay that slammed indiscriminately into her brain. Jealousy moved through her, clutching her stomach and shoving shame into her chest. She leaned against the sink behind the bar and breathed. It wasn't that she was jealous of Fay being with Max that way. No, it wasn't that. Grace was damned sure he'd had plenty of women in his time—the man couldn't help being devastatingly attractive.

It was the thought of his being with a woman who could satisfy him, who could give him a night he wouldn't forget, a woman who wouldn't cry when he tried to touch her intimately, or freeze when he held her down. A woman who would ride him with abandon, take control, and allow him to do the same. She was envious of Fay and the unadulterated sex that burst from her and the way in which she embraced it without apology.

It was so unfair. It was unfair that one man, a man she'd trusted, loved, worshipped even, had stripped her of all the sexual confidence she'd ever had. He stole it from her violently, possessively, and beat her with it, leaving scars inside and out.

No.

Grace knew she could never match up to a woman like Fay.

And it hurt.

It hurt all over again.

•   •   •

Max knew there was something wrong with Grace even before they started their run the following morning. She seemed so far away, lost in her head, leaving her unnervingly quiet. He'd asked if she was okay as they stretched, and she'd answered that she was fine, but he wasn't convinced. She looked . . . sad. The green of her eyes was less emerald as though dulled by her thoughts.

They ran their route the same as they always did, stopped for water, and carried on. There was no exclaiming about colors or the beauty of the forest, as there was ordinarily from Grace. She didn't even rummage around in her bra and pull out her phone to take any pictures, which had become, arguably, the highlight of Max's day.

Shit was not okay.

He slowed down to a quick walk, waiting for her to realize that and join him, which she did with a curious expression.

"Are you all right?" she asked, looking him over and trying to spot an injury.

"I'm good," he answered. "I was just thinking, maybe we could change it up a little today. I know another way that we haven't used yet."

She glanced around and shrugged. "Okay."

He set off, leaving the dirt path and heading farther into the forest, knowing the track he'd explored as a kid like the back of his hand, jumping over fallen trees, over puddles left from the overnight rain, and dodging the thick branches that tried to grab them as they ran. It was darker the deeper they ventured; the sun blocked by the canopy of leaves, making it cooler, more eerie.

"Max," Grace panted at his side. "Where the hell are we going?"

"Just wait," he called back. "Come on."

They ran for a few more minutes before, with a yell, Grace came to a grinding halt, breathless and sweating, her eyes darting about the place.

"Where are you taking me, Max?" she demanded, shifting from foot to foot. "I have no idea where we are! This isn't funny."

With any other half-dressed, hot woman alone with him in the woods, Max would have made a joke about being a kidnapper eager to have his wicked way with her. But something in her tone, the anxious shake of her voice, warned him that that probably wasn't a good idea.

He held up his palms. "It's all right. We're almost there. Look."

He turned and pointed through the trees where sunlight and the faint sound of running water filtered through. Max watched Grace carefully. He saw the tension in her neck, the cautiousness in her face, and was immediately contrite. They were still only getting to know each other and here he was, a drug addict, leading her into the deep, dark forest. No wonder she was freaking out.

"Shit. I didn't mean to alarm you or anything. I just wanted to show you something."

Grace regarded him for a moment before she rubbed a hand down her face and exhaled noisily. "No. *I'm* sorry. I'm— It's not you. I just . . . ignore me."

Max nodded. "It's just through there."

Grace lifted her hand. "Lead the way."

Max did as she asked, steering her through more underbrush before, with a push of branches, they emerged into a clearing punctuated by tall trees and blanketed with small yellow flowers, which bobbed in the breeze. The stream ran almost straight through the far end, filling the area with the sounds of splashes, and gurgling, as it dropped down the hill they'd climbed.

Grace gasped at his side. "What is this place?" Her gaze fixed on what remained of a one-room stone cottage, its windows, door, and roof eaten by the elements and looking like something out of a Disney fairy tale.

"Isn't it great?" Max asked. "I found it when I was here on vacation with my dad. I think everyone forgot about it along with your place." He pointed into the distance. "Which is only ten minutes that way."

Her eyes widened, the familiar sparkle returning. "You're kidding?"

Max chuckled. "I thought you'd like it, you know; take some cool pictures or whatever." He rubbed the back of his neck, the realization of doing something nice for another person prickling his skin with unfamiliarity.

Her hand brushed his forearm. "It's incredible."

Grace wandered through the flowers and trees, touching them, exploring the ruins, and dipping her feet into the stream. Max sat on an overturned log, drinking his water, watching her and smiling as her contagious delight crept back. He grinned when she made a song and dance about pulling her cell phone from her bra, and took photo after photo, promising herself she'd return with her Nikon. He leaned back on the heels of his hands, lifting his face to the warm May sunshine and allowed the calm and quiet to soak into his bones.

"Do you find me attractive?"

Max frowned before he opened one eye. "I'm sorry, what?"

Grace stood by the stream, arms loose at her sides, looking more than a little uncomfortable. "Do you find me attractive, yes or no?"

Opening both eyes, Max cleared his throat. "Is this a trick?"

"Not a trick."

Max didn't feel all that assured. "It sounds like a trick."

"We're friends, right?"

He sat forward, resting his elbows on his bare knees. "Um, I guess."

"Okay, good. I'd like you to be honest with me."

Max exhaled with a disbelieving chuckle. "I'm not sure I can answer your question without saying *something* wrong."

He knew how women worked. She'd find at least one thing in his answer she didn't like the sound of. Plus, he didn't want to come across as a sexist pig, which he was bound to do, looking at her in her running gear, all innocent face and beautiful glistening skin.

Grace approached him. "Okay. Let me ask you another way. Would you have sex with me?"

Now *that* question Max's body undoubtedly paid attention to. He was suddenly glad his shorts were loose. Shit. He shifted where he sat. "What? Are you— Why are you asking me this?"

She shrugged. "Just curious." She crossed her arms. "It's okay if you don't. I get it."

Max barked out a laugh. "My God. Women! I didn't even answer and you've already assumed the worst."

"Well, I'm not like Fay from the bar," she argued. "So I can see why you wouldn't want me that way; the way you wanted her."

Her words weren't petulant or bitter, there was no hint of jealousy. She was resigned, accepting of what she thought was true, and it stopped Max short. How could she believe the shit she was spouting?

He stood and took two steps toward her. "No," he agreed. "You're nothing like Fay. And thank God for that." Surprise lightened her eyes. "And just so we're clear," he added. "I didn't want her and I didn't have sex with her."

Grace blinked. "You didn't?"

Max shook his head. "I wouldn't believe everything you hear."

"But she's so sexual," Grace uttered. "And her boobs are amazing." She looked genuinely puzzled.

Max snorted. "That she is, but, firstly, I was far too fuckin' drunk. And, secondly, for a guy, all boobs are amazing, especially when they have Apple logos creased on 'em."

He knew how flirtatious his comment was, but the laugh that exploded out of Grace made his unease worth it.

"Where is this comin' from?" he asked with a lift of his shoulders. "I thought we were cool just like this." Max knew that if she wanted more from him, he needed to put the brakes on whatever they were doing, pronto.

"We are," Grace insisted. "Oh, God, this is great." She waved her hand between them and then to their surroundings. "I love running with you, and hanging out, it's just . . ."

Max waited, seeing the indecision skirt across her mouth.

She had a great mouth.

He fidgeted.

"Look," he offered, sensing the odd curve their friendship was about to take. "I wanna be straight with you: I'm nowhere near in a position to offer *any* woman a relationship. I'm fucked up. I have serious attachment and trust issues. I'm a drug addict. I'm fighting every day to stay in recovery, and getting involved with someone wouldn't be fair to either of us."

A small V punctuated Grace's brow. "Who said anything about a relationship? I was talking about sex."

Max laughed and clutched the bridge of his nose. "Fair enough." He leveled her with a stare. "But I still wouldn't have sex with you." The red-blooded male in him immediately smacked him upside the head with a what-the-fuck-dude? Before Grace could look even more despondent, he admitted, "I find you very, very attractive."

"You do?"

"You own a mirror, right?"

She smiled faintly. "But you still wouldn't—"

"Because you deserve better than that," he interrupted. "You deserve more than some asshole like me who can offer you nothing but an emotionless fuck. You deserve someone who'll take you out and treat you right." He shook his head. "I can't do that. I'm not capable of that right now." He swallowed down the regret. "I don't think I'll ever be capable of that again."

Grace stared at him for a moment, searching his face for answers to fill in the blanks of his past. Her gaze did funny things to Max's chest. "Okay. Thank you for being honest with me," she murmured. "I appreciate it."

He dipped his chin. "Sure."

She rubbed her hands together and set off toward the direction of her house. "But now at least I know who to come to for an emotionless fuck, right?"

Max grinned at the exaggerated sway of her ass and hips.

Fucking woman.

· · · ·

Whiskey's was busier than Max had seen since he'd arrived in town. Ruby's coworker Buck was celebrating his thirtieth birthday, and she'd invited Max to join them. It had been a few weeks since he'd shattered his sober streak, and he'd avoided the bar and the careful invitations that his friends and family offered him ever since, but, besides being a stubborn son of a bitch, he knew he couldn't delay the inevitable any longer. As it was, he liked the atmosphere of the place, he liked the people who frequented it, and he enjoyed spending downtime with his uncle. The banter with him and the awesome food undoubtedly took his mind off the temptations behind the bar.

His gaze slid over to Grace, who was popping the cap off a bottle of beer for a customer, and he cleared his throat.

Too fucking tempting.

Eager to distract himself, Max sat with his cousin, her husband, and their friends and listened to them reminisce about Buck as a kid, his less than stellar behavior at school, and his obsession with *Star Wars*.

Max listened, adding anecdotes about Ruby as a teenager and receiving smacks of embarrassment from her, much to the delight of Uncle Vince, who elaborated with gusto. Max sipped his orange juice, smiled at the stories he heard, and tried not to wonder why his gaze continually kept traveling back to the bar, where Grace was working hard, smiling as she served beer and food, and generally looking lovely.

It had been two days since she'd asked him about whether he found her attractive, and for two days he'd been chewing it over. It sure came out of left field, although, in hindsight, it shouldn't have been surprising after he'd left the bar with Fay draped all over him.

He hated that he'd done that.

He hated that Grace believed she was less attractive than Fay—who was watching him predatorily from her seat near the pool table—and he was truly perplexed that Grace wasn't aware of how hot she was. As much as he maintained his sexual distance, keeping their relationship as platonic as possible, Max wasn't immune to the way Grace looked.

Jesus.

A year ago, he wouldn't have given a shit about her feelings, his feelings, or anything else for a chance to get her into bed, against a wall, in the backseat of his car, on his desk in the body shop office, but now things were different.

Since rehab, he had feelings about this shit. He knew Grace had feelings and, as much as she assured him that all she wanted from him was sex, he knew that no woman was that black and white. There were always areas of gray where someone got hurt; someone was left disappointed. Max had been that guy, moving from one piece of ass to the next with no regard for how they felt or who he was hurting. He fucked to forget and in doing so, he forgot what his bed partners felt or wanted. He was an asshole.

But he wasn't that man anymore.

Grace was good people. Optimism glowed from her and he couldn't mess with that. Like he'd told her, she deserved more. She deserved to be treated like a queen by a guy who wasn't fucked up, who wasn't always thinking about his next score. She deserved a man to be thinking about *her* 24/7, who made her laugh and smile.

She leaned on the bar as she chatted to Deputy Yates, who, as always, looked like he wanted to ravage her senseless. Prick.

Max pondered. If he could go back two days and answer Grace's question again, would he sleep with her?

Hell yes.

Of course he would.

Damn, he'd fuck her until she screamed. He'd take her in every position he could think of. He'd taste her and make her skin gleam just as it did when they ran. He'd watch her as she came, knowing it would be fucking awesome, and then do it all over again until she begged him to stop. Grace was the kind of woman who deserved to be pleasured hard, pleasured thoroughly—

"You okay over there?" Ruby asked, smirking into the lip of her bottle of beer, knowing full well who Max was looking at.

"Yeah, I'm good," he answered, ignoring her wiggling eyebrows.

Buck snorted. "Of course he's good, he's watching RiRi." He stood up, shaking his ass and slapping it while singing off-key: "Bitch, better have my money!"

Everyone laughed. Ruby rolled her eyes before she snuggled into her husband's side. "You fellas."

"She's smokin', Ruby," Buck stage-whispered as he sat back down. "Am I right, Max?"

Max didn't answer, suddenly finding the toe of his boot fascinating.

"I would wine and dine and slap the hell out of her ass," Buck continued. "And then I'd kiss it better."

Everyone around the table sniggered. It was clear to Max that Buck was perfectly harmless; nevertheless, his words caused a stirring of unease in the depths of Max's belly.

Buck sat up straight, his stare on the bar. "I should ask her out."

"Don't, Buck," Ruby said with a laugh. "You're drunk."

Buck stood, pulling his Black Sabbath T-shirt at the hem in an attempt to look presentable. He ran his hands through his shoulder-length blond hair and made his way, swaying ever so slightly, over to the bar. Max and the entire group of fifteen others watched in hushed silence as Buck smiled at Grace, who smiled back. After a moment, he handed her some money. Grace took it and handed him something in return that looked like a piece of paper. Max kind of hoped it wasn't her phone number. Buck winked at her and walked back to the table.

"What the fuck?" Josh exclaimed.

"That's how you treat a woman, my good man," Buck answered with a smile, folding the piece of paper Grace had given him before wafting it in Josh's face.

Josh coughed a laugh, clearly impressed. "Is that her phone number? Did you actually ask her out?"

Buck dropped back onto his stool, all bravado gone, and lifted the paper. "I tried but then she asked me what I wanted, so"—he opened up the receipt—"I ordered some wings for the table."

Even Max laughed loudly.

.   .   .

It had been a long time since Max had enjoyed himself quite as much, without the help of any illegal substances. He was sober and clean and it felt good; his initial worry about being back in the bar dissolved in the relaxed atmosphere. As the night progressed, Buck got drunker and, the more he drank, the funnier he became. He played rock song after rock song on the jukebox, which Max was all for, and danced on his stool despite being told numerous times to get down and be careful. He tied his belt around his forehead as he performed a stunning and energetic air guitar and shouted every single word to every Led Zeppelin song played.

"He looks like he's having fun," Grace commented as she handed Max another orange juice.

Max smiled, watching Buck prance around the pool table. He danced with each woman he encountered, spinning and twirling them around the place. "He'll have a hell of a sore head tomorrow." He sipped his drink and turned back to Grace, who was on his side of the bar, collecting glasses. "How are you?" he asked.

"Meh. Tired. I'm not sleeping great."

Her eyes widened a little, as though she'd said too much. Max nodded, not wanting to say anything that would make her feel more embarrassed. She grabbed the towel tucked in her waistband and wiped around Max's glass, seemingly agitated about something. He wanted to show he appreciated what suffering from insomnia was like, but wasn't sure how. He didn't want to talk about Lizzie or Christopher despite them being the main reasons he had terrors.

He opened his mouth to speak, to explain that he understood, that he'd listen if she wanted him to, but was interrupted by a large body slamming into his side. A sweaty arm wrapped around his neck along with the stench of beer.

"Maaaaaaaaaaaaax!" Buck held him close. "I knew I'd find you over here with the delectable Grace." Buck pointed to Max. Grace watched them both with a small smile. "He likes you."

"Buck," Max warned, shrugging him off. "Come on, man."

"See!" Buck exclaimed. "He's all embarrassed and shit because he loooooooves you."

Max's cheeks warmed. Whether it was in annoyance or discomfort, he wasn't sure, but the giggle that came from Grace eased it momentarily.

"And why wouldn't he love you, huh?" Buck continued. "You are very pretty."

Grace flushed and dropped her gaze to the floor.

"You are," Buck confirmed, with a small stagger. "I think you're aba—absu—absolutely gorgeous." He took a step toward her. "And you should dance with me because it's my birthday."

"Oh," Grace said, shaking her head and moving backward. "I don't dance."

"Suuure you do!" Buck insisted, moving closer.

She placed her hands up toward Buck's chest and shook her head. "No, I don't, Buck. Come on."

Max saw the panic in Grace's eyes when her back hit the bar. He reached for Buck's forearm. "She doesn't want to."

"Yeah, she does." Buck grabbed Grace's hands and held them fast, swaying with her, and humming. He pulled her to him, wrapping his arms around her, making her look minute against his huge frame.

"Let me go," Grace said, her voice low.

"Oh, come on, one song, honey. One song."

"Buck," Max urged, his hand now on the man's shoulder.

"Please, let me go," Grace said. "You're holding me too tightly. I can't"—she tried to wrench herself from Buck's grasp—"I can't move. I can't breathe."

Buck pulled her away from the bar, twirling around as Max tried to get the bastard's drunk ears to listen.

Grace's eyes closed tightly. "Buck," she said again and wiggled against him.

Buck laughed, his drink-addled mind believing she was having fun.

"Let me go." She tried again to get away from him. Her face crumpled and a shuddering breath filled her lungs. "Buck! Get off me! Get off me, Buck!" The scream of his name ricocheted around the bar. Heads snapped immediately in their direction as Grace fought against the man holding her. "Get off me! Get off me! Now! Now!"

Buck released Grace as though scalded with boiling water, staggering backward into a nearby table, instantly repentant and looking scared to death. After a moment when the whole bar seemed to hold its breath under the fading sounds of Def Leppard, Max reached slowly for Grace. She slapped his hand away. "No. Don't!"

Her shoulders rounded, her knees wobbled, and her eyes scrunched shut, her arms wrapping tightly around herself. Max watched helplessly as her breathing picked up, erratic and shallow, and she screamed that she was having a panic attack.

"Grace," he murmured. "You're okay." She shook her head, trying to breathe. "Grace," Max said again, waving the crowd of concerned regulars away. "Listen, you're safe. No one's going to hurt you. You're safe. Just breathe."

"I'm sorry, Grace," Buck slurred. "I didn't mean to scare you. I was just—"

Deputy Yates, who'd approached from the other end of the bar, touched Grace's shoulder, making her cry out in surprise. Her eyes snapped open, wide and frantic, making Max's breath catch.

What the hell had the poor girl been through?

Her bewildered stare met Max's. "You're all right," he whispered, trying to smile. "Okay?"

She swallowed, her breathing still hurried and gasping. "I—I can't—please?"

Max risked taking a step closer to her. "Tell me what you need."

A sob escaped her throat. She tried to catch it in her shaking hand. "Please, I— Home. Max, please. Take me home. I need to go home."

.   .   .

Grace didn't speak while Max drove her back to the boardinghouse. On hearing her say she needed to get out of the bar, he'd wrapped her in his jacket, knowing the shakes would set in pretty quick, and all but carried her to the truck, ignoring the deputy's pissed expression and his insistence that he should take her.

Dick.

Max glanced over to Grace every minute or so as he drove. Seeing her so small, so scared, and so sad made his chest ache; the woman at his side was a mere shadow of the vibrant, happy Grace he'd come to know. He parked, and turned off the engine. She never moved. He allowed his fingertips to touch her leg. She startled, as he knew she would.

"We're here," he said gently.

She looked out of the window, returning from wherever she'd been in her uncharacteristic silence. She opened the truck door before Max could hurry around the hood and began shuffling across the lot, gripping the edges of his jacket around her hard enough to make her knuckles white. It drowned her, but it was keeping her warm. He followed her up the stairs and along the corridor, thankful that he was only across the hall from her room. If she needed anything, he knew he could get to her quickly. She pulled out her door key, the shaking in her hand pronounced and not conducive to finding a keyhole.

She muttered a curse under her breath before Max took the key and opened the door for her. She entered with a sigh, leaving Max in the doorway, torn. He knew he needed to make sure she was all right to be on her own. She'd knocked back two pills like they were Skittles back at the bar, but he didn't want to freak her out further.

A man making himself at home in her room was not what she needed right now. That shit was clear as day.

"You can come in," she muttered. She turned on the side lamp, kicked off her shoes, and dropped onto the edge of the bed.

Max did as she asked, approaching her cautiously, closing the door behind him. After a moment of silence where she stared at the floor, Grace cupped her palms to her face and began to sob. Carefully, Max crouched in front of her, placing a hand on her arm.

"I'm such an idiot," she managed through her tears. "*Such* an idiot."

"No one thinks that," Max assured her. If anything, everyone in the bar had been terrified by what they saw. Truthfully, he felt sorry for Buck. She'd certainly sobered him up some.

"It's been . . . so long since I've had— I haven't done that for a while. I thought, being here seemed to, I thought it helped me forget."

Max's thumb moved against her skin, a gentle whisper of a movement to calm her. She rubbed her face and wiped inelegantly at her eyes. "I'm so sorry."

"You don't have shit to be sorry about," he told her firmly. "It happens, trust me."

She released a breath of wry laughter. "I guess we're messed up together, huh?"

Max nodded.

Grace closed her bloodshot eyes and exhaled. "I'm just so tired."

"I should let you get some sleep," Max offered, standing gradually and gesturing to her bed.

"That's just it," she complained, slapping her hands to her legs. "I can't. I take my pills and still I lie awake or the nightmares come and I'm too frightened to shut my eyes again." Her face creased, frustration stiffening her shoulders, and the tears started again.

Max rubbed the back of his neck, helpless. "What can I do? Do you want a drink? A bath? I could run you a bath if you want."

Grace sniffed and cleared her throat. "Could you . . . could you stay? Just for a little while. It might help me fall asleep with you here, and I, I don't want to be alone."

The humiliation of asking him such a simple question seemed to wash over her and rest in her imploring eyes.

"Sure," Max said without thought or pause. "Get into bed."

He walked across the room to sit in the high-backed chair in the corner of the room, experiencing a twinge of déjà vu of the day he'd awoken from his own panic attack in rehab to find Elliot watching over him. Grace stayed fully clothed; she didn't even remove Max's jacket. She simply slipped under the covers and snuggled down.

"Thank you, Max," she murmured, her words muffled by the pillow.

"You're welcome."

It took a while for her breathing to even out, for her slight form to lose its hard edges and fall safely into sleep. Strangely, it didn't feel weird for Max to be sitting in the low lamplight watching Grace sleep. It didn't feel imposing or creepy. It felt right. It felt right that she'd asked him and he felt right doing it. He was damn certain he wouldn't have trusted anyone else to do it, especially the asshole cop whose eyes betrayed the lust he harbored for her. Max sat back, comfortable, warm, and he watched. He glanced at the digital clock on Grace's side table.

It was midnight.

He'd stay for another half hour and then he'd leave.

•　•　•

Max was wrenched from an unexpectedly deep sleep by a bloodcurdling scream. Max shot into a sitting position, dazed and shaken, and wondering where the hell he was and what the fuck was going on. Gaining his bearings, Max looked over to the bed to find Grace fighting with the sheets, crying and calling out gibberish that chilled Max's bones. On sleep-heavy legs, he rushed over to the side of the bed. Sweat speckled her grimacing face.

"Grace. You're okay."

Her voice became hoarse with her screams. "Rick, please! Don't, please!"

Max reached for her flailing arms, before she could hurt herself, and took her hands. "Grace, you're safe."

But still she fought.

It wasn't until Max—in a moment of lunacy, and without another solution—climbed into bed with her, holding her close to his chest, that she started to calm. The fight in her ebbed slowly, leaving her breathless, and clutching Max's T-shirt like a lifeline.

"It's okay," he whispered. "I've got you. I won't let him hurt you."

He stroked her hair and whispered words of safety and sleep until she rested once more, her small body clinging to his like a limpet. But that was all right. If a warm body was what she needed, Max was happy to provide it, despite the echo of her screams resonating around the small, dark room. She mumbled and murmured into his neck and Max held her tighter. She moved and shifted and he stroked her hair some more until he, too, was claimed by exhaustion.

15

Max awoke alone. From under a furrowed, tired brow, he glanced around Grace's room, looking for signs of her presence. He called out her name, twice, but there was no reply. With a stretch and a groan, hating the feeling of having slept in his clothes, Max stood from the bed, reaching for the jacket he'd wrapped around Grace the night before. He snuck out, glancing down the hallway, and entered his room.

He needed a long, hot shower and a hard think.

From the moment he and Grace had first met, he'd been in awe of her ability to be so together, so sure and positive. Max had admitted a few weeks ago that he enjoyed spending time with her. Obviously, she was great to look at, but it was more than that. She eased some painful part of him with her stress-free smiles and laughter, and her enthusiasm for almost everything made Max forget the bad shit and focus on the good.

He liked her. He would be happy to call her a friend. And seeing his friend fall apart that way, to see Grace so broken, was hard to take.

Cleaned and dressed, Max headed into the boardinghouse kitchen, where the sounds of Lynyrd Skynyrd and pots clanging alerted Max to his uncle's presence. Vince grinned when he saw Max enter and immediately offered him a freshly buttered piece of toast.

"How's it goin', son?" he asked, throwing a dish towel over his shoulder and stirring a pan of . . . something, which smelled spectacular.

Max spoke around his toast. "Okay. You see Grace this morning?"

Vince's face grew concerned. "She left early. I think she's up at the house. Didn't say much. She okay after last night?"

Max shrugged, wiping his crumby hands on his jeans. "She was pretty spooked." He explained how he'd taken her to her room, but didn't speak a word about her nightmare. That shit was personal. He knew Grace wouldn't appreciate folks knowing that about her and it wasn't for him to tell.

Vince leaned a hip against the kitchen countertop. "Buck's tore up. He was rambling last night about sending her roses, kept asking Caleb if he was gonna get arrested or some shit." A wry smile curved his lips. "I talked him down."

"She knows he was just drunk," Max assured him. "I'm gonna go and see if she's all right." He waved a thumb over his shoulder.

Vince's smile stretched. He nodded. "That's good of you. You tell her, she needs anythin' she just has to ask, okay?"

"I will."

Max drove up to Grace's house, stopping on the way for coffee and muffins, and pulled up in front of what was now a beautiful, clean, freshly painted two-story property. There were still some jobs to complete, the upper-level walls needed plastering, some electrical work, and a few more licks of paint here and there, but it looked amazing.

Max knocked on the front door once before walking in. The way he saw it, until his uncle passed those keys over to Grace, it was still a work site and he was a site worker. Manners be damned. The sounds of "I Heard It Through the Grapevine" drifted from the sitting room. He found Grace sitting cross-legged on the hardwood floor, her hair pulled back, draped in a large hoodie, yoga pants, and sneakers, surrounded by bags and boxes, looking through photographs, the music coming from the cell phone at her side.

He lifted the coffee cups and muffin bag. "I come bearing sustenance."

She raised a hand without looking up. "Shhh, you're stepping on Marvin."

He smiled and approached when she gestured for him to join her on the floor, which he did. He plopped the paper bag close to her.

"Thank you," she uttered. "I knew someone was bound to hear my stomach rumbling eventually."

He lifted the lid of his cup and sipped his mocha. "What are you doin'?" He glanced curiously at the copious amounts of packages.

She sighed and turned off her music. "I ordered some stuff for the house, decorative stuff, and it all arrived today. It completely slipped my mind after . . . well; anyway, I got a phone call at the butt crack of dawn from the deliveryman asking me where the hell I was."

Max frowned. "I never heard your phone."

"You sleep pretty heavy." Grace averted her eyes and opened the muffin bag.

"Apparently."

"Thank you, by the way," she whispered. "For staying with me. I . . . it meant a lot."

"Not a problem. How do you feel?"

She shrugged. "Like a moron. Embarrassed."

Max shook his head. "Don't be. You didn't do anything wrong." A small breath escaped her when she shook her head. "Do you wanna talk about it?" he asked.

She seemed to ponder the offer of a friendly ear before she looked away. "It's a very long, very . . . hard story to tell."

Max picked at his muffin, silently acknowledging her refusal to share. He wasn't sure how to feel about it. He wanted to help her, he wanted to understand, and he wanted to know who the fuck Rick was and what he'd done to her. He wanted to be a friend; he wanted her to trust him.

"You know that Brooks isn't my maiden name, right?" Her words were quiet.

Max nodded. "I heard." Grace bit her bottom lip, fussing with one of the boxes. "Was Rick your husband?" Her head snapped around to him so fast, Max was amazed her eyes didn't wobble out of their sockets.

"What? How do— Why would you ask that?"

"Last night. You called out his name while you were sleeping, like you were scared of him."

Grace's eyes dropped closed before her hand covered her face. "Jesus," she muttered. "I'm so sorry you had to see that, Max. I really am. I—"

"How about you stop apologizing," he insisted with a mouthful of muffin. "Seriously. It's annoying."

A smirk tugged at her mouth. After a quiet moment, she lifted her chin, squared her shoulders, and looked him dead in the eye.

"Yes," she answered. "Rick was my husband."

Max attempted to look indifferent to her confirmation but he wasn't sure he pulled it off. He picked at his muffin, suddenly not very hungry, and waited for her to continue. She didn't. She nursed her drink, not saying a word, leaving the room heavy with expectation. Max shifted under its weight, an alarming thought creeping up his spine.

Maybe she was waiting for him to share, too.

Shit, he didn't know if he could do that. It was bad enough opening up to Elliot, let alone Grace. He glanced over at her while she pulled some brightly colored canvases out of their bags, and he began to appreciate how hard it must have been for her to share even that small slice of information. She *trusted* him; it was only fair he paid her back in kind.

He steeled himself and breathed deeply. "I was engaged once."

Grace stared at him, her mouth dropping open.

"Her name was Lizzie."

There. Tit for tat. Just two friends talking. Sharing. Easy.

The spiking of his pulse suggested otherwise.

"And she broke your heart." Grace's statement floated around them like dark, thunderous clouds, conjuring a sharp nod from Max as reply. It was all he could do, his throat blocked by too many words.

"Rick and I got engaged when my mother passed away."

Max looked at her, recognizing Grace's familiar strength ripple beneath the surface. He dipped his chin for her to continue.

"My brother, Kai, never liked him, said he was trouble, but . . . I was madly in love. We'd been together for eighteen months after meeting at the bar I worked in, and I was ready to be his wife." She pushed the bags and boxes away, held her latte close, and spoke toward the floor. "The wedding was small but Rick treated me like a princess. We bought an apartment; we talked about children, the whole nine yards. I was sickeningly happy."

Max moved closer, their shoulders just touching. "What changed?"

She smiled sadly. "He got a promotion at work and . . . nothing was ever the same again." She pulled her knees up to her chest. "Before we were married, Rick would always tell me how beautiful I was, how lucky he was to have such an amazing-looking wife. He liked showing me off and I liked him doing it. It made me feel good about myself having a husband who desired me." Her cheeks darkened at the admission.

"He worked in advertising, had since college, long hours, and mammoth workload. He partied as hard as he worked, but it never occurred to me to mind. That was just Rick. He was the life and soul. That's what attracted me to him. Finally, after months of barely seeing each other, he got a promotion to head an important deal. He was over the moon. To celebrate there was an office party. I bought a new dress. I wanted to look special for him, pretty for him, so he could be proud to have me at his side." She paused. "Looking back, I think I bought it because I knew something wasn't right. He'd become distant, moody, less attentive, but I put it down to the amount of work he had. While working for the promotion, he'd started drinking every night. There was always a bottle of something on the kitchen counter when I got up in the mornings."

Max turned his body toward her.

"All night at the party, Rick's work colleagues commented about what a fine couple we were, how lucky Rick was to have me, how lovely I looked. He thanked them and smiled, but it never reached his eyes." She pulled her knees closer and sighed. "Anyway, when we got home from the party, Rick accused me of flirting with his coworkers, of embarrassing him. I called him crazy and delusional and he pushed me against the wall, telling me I needed to learn some respect . . ." She blew out a long breath between pursed lips. "He wasn't gentle."

Max's stomach rolled. "Christ, Grace."

"I didn't know the man who pinned me to the wall. He was a stranger. The entire time he told me I was a tease, how I'd humiliated him by looking like a slut, how I'd loved all the attention being on me and not him." She rubbed her hands down her face. "It was only later I found out he wasn't just drunk but high"—she looked at Max—"on cocaine."

Max blinked, knowing he shouldn't have been surprised, but he was startled all the same. "Fuck." He dropped his head, his chin tapping his chest.

"He'd gotten involved with some guys he'd met through work and started using heavily to cope with the stress after his promotion. He kept it a secret from me. He'd use it to keep awake so he could meet deadlines. Later I discovered he'd been a heavy user in college, too, before we met. Every night it became the same: he'd go out, get shitfaced, high, come home, and take it out on me."

"Why did you stay with him?" Max asked, desperate to keep

the incredulity from his voice, because who the fuck was he to judge about making bad decisions?

"I tried, but he would apologize," Grace answered too matter-of-factly for Max's taste. "He'd promise me he'd change, beg for another chance. He'd take me out; make love to me as I remembered. He'd go back to being like the man I fell in love with, the man I married, for a day or two and then . . ."

"And then he'd hit you."

Grace's face was all the answer he needed.

"I hope the fucker is rotting in a prison cell somewhere," Max growled, running his hands through his hair.

"He's on parole, living in the apartment we bought back in California." The unspoken question must have been a beacon on Max's face. "He served two years in state prison for assault and battery after he shattered my hip, collapsed my lung, and broke three of my ribs the night I told him I was leaving him."

Revulsion heaved through Max. So much about Grace now made sense. Her aching injury when they ran, her abhorrent fear of Buck and his behavior, and the subsequent panic attack and nightmare. Her continuing wariness of Deputy Cock's advances and flirting, her desperate need to be independent, to show that fucker ex-husband of hers she could be in control of her life, in the face of what he did to her.

In spite of what she'd suffered at the hands of a man who should have been worshipping her body and loving her, she was moving on, being strong, finding the good in shit Max didn't even notice or pay attention to. His respect for the woman at his side multiplied exponentially.

What it didn't explain, however, was why she wanted to be close to Max. Why did she want to be friends with a recovering drug addict when she'd suffered so much at the hands of another? Was it a test for her? Was it simply for her own recovery, or did she really want to know him?

"I know what you're thinking," Grace murmured. "And you're wrong. You're nothing like him. Nothing, believe me."

Max scoffed and leaned his forearms on his bent knees. "We're all the fucking same," he answered despondently, his eyes on the floor between his feet. "Addicts. Our brains are wired identically. We want the same things and we don't give a shit who we hurt to get it."

"Did you beat up the woman you loved, rape her, abuse her with words so vile you'd pray for silence?"

"No," Max replied firmly, offended by her question. "I'd never fucking— I loved her, I'd . . . Never."

Grace smiled sadly. "See. Nothing alike."

Max's hands found his hair again. "It's not that black and white, Grace. I may not have done those things, but I've done my fair share of fucked-up shit. Shit I'm not proud of, stuff that I'm still working through." He exhaled heavily. "You shouldn't want to have anything to do with me."

"I'm a big girl," she retorted. "I can make that decision for myself."

Max wasn't so sure. The urge to bolt, to save her from his past, his addiction, his mistakes, swelled in his stomach, but for the life of him, he couldn't lift himself up off the floor.

"Do you know what I saw when I looked at my husband the last time in that courtroom?" Grace asked. "I saw hate. I saw violent anger and a monster unleashed by all the drugs and all the drinking. I saw secrets, threats. I saw a man who was seconds away from self-destruction, a man who, had the police not been called by a neighbor who heard my screaming, would have killed me. There wasn't even a shadow of the man I married." She nudged his shoulder. "Do you know what I see when I look at you?"

Max shook his head fervently. "I'd rather not know—"

"I see a man who wants so much to be better, who regrets the decisions he made, who wants to make amends and move on with his life. I see a man terrified to take a chance, to trust, but desperate to do so. I see a man who's fractured, but trying. I see hope."

He looked at her askance, too stunned to speak, too wary to believe her.

"You're a good man, Max," she said, standing with a groan and wiping the dust off her ass with her hands. "Now stop overthinking things and help me with these boxes."

And just like that, the conversation was over.

•　　•　　•

Grace's head was still groggy. It always was the day after an attack. It was like swimming through wet concrete. Her whole body was heavy and stiff, but she wouldn't let it slow her down, not when she had her new home to make beautiful. She looked over at Max, balancing on a ladder he'd fetched from his uncle, hanging a large canvas on her wall. An expression of concentration on his handsome face.

Waking up next to Max that morning had been a surprise, to say the very least. A good surprise, but a surprise nonetheless. She'd woken with a headache evil enough to cripple a rhino, dazed and unable to move. Max's forearm had been wrapped tightly around her waist, his strong chest to her back, his nose in the crook of her neck. He was an epic big spoon.

She hadn't even remembered him getting into bed with her, but her heart warmed at his thoughtfulness. He was more caring and compassionate than he realized. Even his arriving with a latte and muffin for her was something he probably didn't give a second's thought about. He was so used to playing the role of the big bad wolf that he couldn't see how good he actually was. Sure, he still had a lot to work through—Grace wasn't that naïve—but he was so much more than he gave himself credit for.

"Is this good?" he called out, holding the canvas against the wall, his large arms open wide, the red T-shirt he was wearing pulling deliciously across his broad shoulders.

Grace crossed her arms over her chest, admiring the view. "Um, a little to the left." He did as she asked. "A little to the right." Again, he complied. "Up." He sighed. "Down."

"Grace."

"Now left. Right." She was giggling into her fist as he turned to glare at her.

"Are you fucking kidding me?"

"Oh, come on, lighten up," she said with a wave of her hand.

"I'll lighten up when you make a damned decision," he grumbled, but Grace wasn't blind to the small smile he tried to hide.

"Where you had it was perfect."

He mumbled to himself and set about hammering in the hooks to hold it. They'd blown off their usual run—both of them too tired after the prior evening's frivolities—and, with neither of them working, had set about putting up the pictures, mirrors, and art pieces Grace had bought. Max hadn't questioned her when she'd asked for help and had worked diligently all afternoon, even driving into town to get them lunch.

His laid-back attitude and his unquestionable acceptance of her life story endeared him even more to her. It had been a long time since she'd opened up to someone new, someone who wasn't family or getting paid to listen, but it hadn't been as difficult as she'd supposed. Max listened intently, as he always did. She saw no pity in his large, dark eyes, only anger and alarm and, predictably, guilt.

But that was simply ridiculous. He could argue all he liked—and she didn't doubt he would—but Grace knew and her gut knew: Max was good to his bones. She didn't know why he'd gotten embroiled in drugs, although his mentioning of his fiancée may have been a clue. But she saw he was nothing like Rick.

Nothing.

She hummed while she hung another picture. A fraying piece of fabric stamped with the Martin Luther King quote, "We must accept finite disappointment, but never lose infinite hope." It had been her mother's favorite and it took pride of place in the hallway. It would be the first thing her guests would see when they walked into the house.

She stood back, liking its placement, suddenly aware that there was no noise coming from Max's part of the room. She turned to find him watching her, an intense expression on his face, his arms folded.

"What?" she asked.

"Is that why you asked me? Because of what he did to you?"

Grace frowned. "Asked you?"

"The other day, on our run, about whether I found you attractive, about whether I'd have sex with you. Is it because of what he did?"

Ah. That.

Grace's cheeks warmed. "Kind of." She exhaled. "It's a little more complicated than that."

Max remained silent, expectant.

"I've tried being with a man twice since Rick and both times were disasters."

And that was putting it mildly. Her first attempt ended with a trip to the ER, Grace unable to breathe for the flashbacks that began hammering her when he'd climbed on top of her. Her second was equally heinous.

She approached Max slowly. "I couldn't handle them . . . being on—holding me down; holding me too tightly. Truthfully, I struggled with everything intimate. It didn't take my therapist to explain why."

"So why would me touching you be any different?" Max asked his brow creasing.

Grace smiled. "Because you're the first guy since my husband that I've wanted to get close to. Not like that," she explained when he fidgeted uncomfortably. "I wanted to get to know you, be your friend. I felt safe being near you, and the urge to run away and lock myself in a room goes away when we hang out." Grace cleared her throat, awkwardness teasing her neck. "I just thought that . . . because I can handle being with you, I might be able to handle being *with* you."

Max's eyes widened when understanding struck. "I see."

Grace toed the floor with her bare foot. "You saw what happened when Buck touched me. You think I want that to happen the rest of my life every time someone wants to fool around?" Anger bubbled through her. "I hate that *he* has power over me, even when we've been apart all this time. I hate that *he* still gets to dictate who I can be with, who I can be friends with. He doesn't deserve that power. He did nothing to earn it."

"I agree. You shouldn't let him control your life."

"I want to reclaim it." Her voice raised in volume. "I want to be sexy again. I want to be passionate, and not afraid to be sexual."

Their eyes met for a brief moment, until Max looked away with a deep inhalation. He rubbed his face. The sound of his whiskers scratching his palm did funny things to Grace's belly.

"Can I be honest with you?" he asked, his expression sincere but torn.

"Of course you can."

He paused, opening his mouth a number of times without speaking. He stretched his neck and shifted his weight. "You're hot, all right," he said finally. "And you're sexy as all hell; you really shouldn't worry about that. And six months ago, I would have fucked you any way you wanted me to." He stared. "Shit, I'd *still* fuck you any way you wanted me to."

Grace swallowed. "Okay."

"But, like I said, you deserve more than that."

"I don't want more than that, Max," she argued. He appeared doubtful. Grace stepped forward. "All right," she began. "Hypothetically, if you agreed to this, what would be your terms, your limits?"

"'This' being us fucking?" Max clarified.

"Yes."

He lifted his chin, his eyes traveling down her body in a way that caused her skin to heat. "No cuddling, no lovey-dovey talk, no pet names, no kissing."

Grace cocked her head. "No kissing, period, or . . ."

"On the mouth," he answered quietly. "It's too intimate."

Grace smirked. "How very *Pretty Woman* of you."

"Pretty what?"

She waved her hand. "Never mind. Those seem fair terms."

Even the cuddling. She wasn't about to tell him how he'd held her all night long. That would be her little secret.

"No promises, no expectations," he added, firmly counting the limits on his fingers. "We use a condom." He pointed at her, his expression grave. "That's a deal breaker for me."

"Of course. I'd expect nothing less." She watched Max gather himself. "Anything else?"

He pressed his lips together. "I don't think so. As long as we're clear that this is what it is, nothing more. We're friends. No relationship, no love, no bullshit."

Bitterness laced every word, but Grace nodded anyway. "Sure. You're just a friend helping me move forward," she said as though reading from a textbook. "We try it once and see what happens, right?"

"Right."

"Okay." Grace licked her lips, underlying excitement pinging through her veins.

Max cleared his throat and shifted where he stood. "And if you're not okay the first time?"

Grace lifted a shoulder, praying to everything she adored that she would be. She'd be mortified if she had another attack in front of Max. "Then we can try again," she offered, her voice lifting as though it was a question. She didn't want to assume Max would want to sleep with her more than once, despite his words to the contrary. "Until I can handle being touched without freaking out like an idiot and I find someone who can love me, warts, and all, we do this."

She smiled, but Max didn't reciprocate. She understood his reticence, of course; this was a big deal; but Grace didn't allow herself to worry about how their being intimate might throw a wrench into the workings of their friendship. He'd made it abundantly clear where he stood, and Grace would respect that. Plus she trusted herself not to let any nonplatonic feelings creep into the equation. No. She wouldn't. It was what it was. No more.

She looked Max square in the eye. "It won't get weird. Promise."

"Good." His shoulders dropped slightly; he was apparently relieved. "What about you?" he asked after a beat of silence. "What're your limits?"

She blinked at him, surprised by his question.

"Grace, I don't want to touch you and make you panic," he added steadily. "If this is gonna work, you have to tell me what I can and can't do."

Grace licked her lips and thought hard about what *would* make her panic, what would scare her. Looking at Max so earnest and responsible, she struggled to bring anything to mind.

"I . . . don't like being held down," she said gently, recollecting the previous night. "As you saw with Buck, I can't handle being— I get claustrophobic." She pulled her hair over her shoulder. "I need to be able to move my hands."

"Understood. What else?"

Her heart skipped as a memory of her and Rick flashed through her psyche. His angry voice, her tears, his hands on her head holding her to his body. "This may be another deal breaker for you." She closed her eyes, not wanting to see Max's face while she spoke. "I don't, I can't . . . go down—I don't like it." She opened her eyes slowly. Max's expression hadn't changed. "He wasn't— Rick wasn't kind when I did it . . ."

A muscle in Max's jaw jumped and his gaze burned hot. "I get it," he said softly. "And I can live with that." He paused before the corner of his mouth lifted wolfishly. "Do you like it being done to you?"

Grace coughed. "I, um, I don't—I can, um, yeah, I don't mind."

Max laughed, his face regaining its usual gentleness. "Good to know."

Grace chuckled, too. The tension in the room lifted around them. "So, are we gonna do this?"

His grin dropped. "As long as you know that I can't give you any more than—"

"It's just sex. I get it," Grace interrupted with mock exasperation. "Seriously, dude, you're not *that* hot. You'd think you had a whole gaggle of women following you around declaring their undying love!"

Max barked out a laugh, his cheeks pinking adorably. He rubbed the back of his neck, a nervous gesture to which Grace was becoming accustomed.

She stuck out her hand. "Shall we shake on it, just to make sure there's no misunderstanding? That we're just two friends helping each other out." Confusion flitted across Max's face. "Oh, please." Grace laughed. "You need this as much as I do. I don't care what you say." He narrowed his gaze but didn't respond. "Deal?" she asked.

He looked from her eyes to her hand and back again, before he took it and squeezed gently. "Deal."

16

"You seem tense," Elliot noted as he wrote on his legal pad.

Max shifted under his shrink's all-knowing stare.

"You wanna tell me about it?"

"Not really."

The truth was, since Max had decided to help Grace with her . . . intimacy problem, he'd been feeling all sorts of chaotic. The day after the deal was agreed to, Grace left for DC. Following her panic attack, she'd arranged an emergency appointment with her therapist. She also wanted to spend a little time with her brother, which suited Max just fine.

A bit of space before the inevitable could only be a good idea, right?

He exhaled heavily and clasped the bridge of his nose. Seriously, he was losing his damned mind if he thought he needed space from Grace. If anything, he'd missed seeing her the two days she was away. His run wasn't nearly as fun on his own. It wasn't space he needed. It was the chance to contemplate what their agreement meant. And after he'd contemplated, ruminated, and brooded like the motherfucker he was for forty-eight hours, he conceded that the mere thought of fucking Grace left him in a cold sweat.

It was crazy. He'd had sex before, for Christ's sake. *A lot* of sex before, and he'd never analyzed it as much as he had for the last seven days. He'd had women of all ages, sizes, and races, and enjoyed them, but Grace was different. Things with Grace were different. She wasn't some broad he'd picked up in a bar and never thought about seeing again. She was a friend.

Once Grace had returned from DC, looking and sounding more relaxed, they'd fallen back into their old routine. They ran, talked, and hung out at her house, even when Max wasn't working. He helped her paint, hung more pictures, and even took her to the local garden center to look at plants she wanted for the place. Things were just as they'd been before she left, except, they weren't. Because, in all the time they'd spent together since they'd shaken hands, neither one of them had made a move.

Not one.

Not a light touch, a lingering glance, or even a fuck it, let's get down to it.

Nothing.

Max had thought about it. Jesus, how he'd thought about it. He'd watched her work behind the bar, and he'd watched her run, but now he imagined what it would be like to touch her under that skirt she wore at Whiskey's, or even taste the sweat that trickled down the sides of her face as they ran. He listened to her laugh, watched her throw her head back, and wondered if she'd do the same when she came.

Yeah, "tense" was a great word for it. It'd been a long time since his cock had taken such an active role in his day-to-day life. Ever since his body recognized Grace as no longer off-limits, it had been more than willing to "help" her out whenever she needed.

"Are your meds working? Any more terrors?"

Max began nibbling the corner of his thumbnail. He shook his head in answer to Elliot's question, pondering whether he should simply tell all about Grace. He knew what the doctor's first instinct would be. He'd think Max was getting involved in a relationship, which he wasn't, and he'd explain how it was a bad idea.

Maybe it *was* a bad idea. But seeing Grace's face as she told him about what she'd been through and the struggles she still dealt with daily was all the push he needed to help her. She wanted to win, to reclaim herself from that fucker who beat her, and who was Max to deny her?

"I have a question," he blurted around his hand. "A hypothetical."

Elliot's brows jumped. "I'm all ears."

"Okay, so," Max began, sitting forward. "Relationships for recovering addicts are a bad thing, right?"

"Not an altogether bad thing, no, but we try to *dissuade* patients from engaging in any new romantic attachments. The emotions can be too overwhelming at the beginning of a relationship and have been known to trigger a relapse."

Max clasped his hands together and let them fall between his knees. "And what about sex? Do you dissuade your patients from that, too?"

Elliot paused, his hand by his face, the pen between his fingers motionless. "As long as you're safe and honest with your partner, I don't see anything wrong with your having sex."

"Why do I feel like there's a 'but' comin'?" Max asked wryly.

Elliot placed his legal pad on the arm of his chair. Uh-oh. "I simply want to make sure you're not substituting one need for another, Max."

"It's not like that, Doc," he said vaguely. "She's . . . we're not— It's complicated."

Elliot nodded but didn't push. "And she knows about your past, your addiction?"

"Some. She knows about my rehab, you, Tate. I've mentioned Lizzie."

"That's good, Max." His smile was proud. "That's a good start. Honesty in *any* relationship, platonic or otherwise, is vitally important."

Yeah, that much Max knew. He sat back in his seat, feeling somewhat calmer with Elliot's affirmation that sex was okay—not that Max wouldn't have done it anyway if he'd said no. He *was* the biggest rule breaker and asshole there was, after all. But his therapist's words eased an anxious part of him that had been griping for more than a week.

The drive back from his session was long. Max wound the window of his truck down and enjoyed the warm evening air on his face, allowing it to help build up the resolve that had started to take shape while sitting in Elliot's office. The whole thing with Grace would become problematic only if he allowed it to. He'd opened up to her and shared things that, ordinarily, would have had him disappearing inside himself. That was the hard bit out of the way.

Sex was easy. Sex he knew. Sex he was good at. Sex with Grace would no doubt be awesome.

He just needed to, as Grace would say, stop overthinking it, and by the time he pulled up outside the boardinghouse, he had. He was going to fuck a hot woman with no strings attached. Any other normal guy would be singing from the rooftops and it was about time he did the same. He smacked his hands on the steering wheel, resolute.

No pressure, no worries, no fuss.

Yeah, he was going to start enjoying himself, goddamn it.

•   •   •

Tate arrived the following morning with his customary wide smile and a yellow T-shirt decorated with—

"What the fuck is that?" Max asked with a puzzled shake of his head, once they'd sat down in their usual seat in the coffee shop, each having bought a sub sandwich.

Tate glanced down at himself and cocked an eyebrow. "It's a Minion dressed as Wolverine," he answered, his tone clearly disgusted with Max's lack of comic book expertise. "What the hell else would it be?"

Max snorted. "I apologize. I'm obviously having an off day with DC—"

"Marvel! Jesus."

"Whatever."

Tate shook his head, looking out of the window toward the sky, his mouth full of sandwich. "I don't even know why I keep coming back to see you. I really don't."

"Because you love me," Max retorted, taking a mammoth bite of his chicken on rye.

Tate shrugged. "Someone has to, I guess." They sat in companionable silence, watching the world go by, while they ate. "So how have things been?"

Max nodded. "Okay. Got my six-month medallion."

Never for one moment had Max thought he'd get to that point, but the gold medal in his pocket proved it. When he'd been awarded it at his last group session, it had been the first time he'd truly felt a shiver of pride.

Tate grinned. "My man. Nice." They fist-bumped. "Any more 'off' days?"

Max shook his head. He and Tate stayed in contact a lot of the time, exchanging texts at least once a day, sometimes more, with phone calls just as regular. Since Max's drunken shenanigans, Tate had been a true crutch for him. The fact that the man traveled to Preston County every week to see Max was testament to how he viewed his role as Max's sponsor.

As they always did, they shot the shit about therapy, caught up on friends, and drank coffee. With Riley at the helm, Max's body shop was booming, and Carter was stressed with Kat's wedding planning. Without warning, and with his hand wrapped around his coffee cup frozen in midair, Tate's attention suddenly diverted from Max to something on the street. Max followed his line of sight and smirked.

It was Grace.

Dressed in her running gear and sweating gorgeously, she was walking down the main road toward the coffee shop, playing with her wristwatch, no doubt checking her run time, which she always did. Her hair was pulled back, her ponytailed curls bouncing, her running pants breathtakingly tight. Max's cock gave a nod of appreciation for those bad boys. He was pissed he'd had to cancel his run with her this morning.

"Good Lord," Tate muttered, gawking at her through the window and spinning around to watch her enter the shop.

"Like what you see?" Max asked around the lip of his cup. A curious and unfamiliar warmth crept across his skin as he observed his sponsor stare at Grace.

"Yeah, um . . . Shit, do they all look like her around here?"

Max looked over at Grace, catching her eye. She beamed and waved. He dipped his chin back at her. "No," he answered.

Just as Max predicted, Grace, with latte and muffin in hand, sauntered across the shop toward them. "Hey," she greeted, her green eyes dancing.

"Hey yourself. Good run?"

"Yeah. Weirdly boring without you." Her gaze darted to Tate. "Hello, you must be Tate, Max's sponsor. I've heard a lot about you."

Tate held out his hand, which Grace took nervously. "All good things, I hope." He grinned, wide and toothy. Max rolled his eyes.

Grace laughed. "Oh, yeah, all good things."

Tate's head snapped to Max. Max sighed. "This is Grace," he introduced. Tate's eyebrows rose. "She's my running partner."

"Running partner, huh?" The expression on Tate's face highlighted how full of bullshit he thought Max to be. But hell, he could think what he liked.

"Yes," Grace said. "You interrupted an important run today." Her playful expression was lovely and Max watched Tate fall headfirst for its captivating powers.

"Well, we can't have that, can we?" Tate played along. "Maybe I can buy you a coffee to make it up to you."

Max cleared his throat and crossed his arms, his attention on the street outside because, well, shit, he didn't know where to look while his sponsor hit on his . . . friend.

"Thank you, but I have my latte already," Grace answered, lifting the cup.

In the glass of the window, Max could see her reflection. Her face, smiling, but timid. He wasn't about to step in, though, not unless she looked to be truly freaking out. Besides, Tate was harmless. An asshole, but harmless all the same.

"Hey, Max," she said suddenly, bringing his gaze back. "Could you meet me at the cottage by the stream later? I'm working through lunch at the bar but I can be there for three thirty." She seemed nervous.

"Should I be worried?"

"Oh, no. I just need your help with something."

"I'll be there."

She smiled, the reticence fading. "Great. It was nice meeting you, Tate."

"The pleasure was all mine, Grace." Tate's eyes never left her until she disappeared down the street.

Max waited with bated breath.

"Okay," Tate ordered with an index finger pressed into the table. "Fucking spill. Who is she and why the hell haven't you talked about her before? And don't give me any of that running partner bullshit. She's hot for you and if you aren't hitting that, I'm revoking your man card right fucking now."

Max laughed despite himself. "She's not hot for me. It's not like that."

Tate gaped, mouth and palms open, looking too much like his brother, Riley. "She's so hot for you, how can you— Look, whatever. Why are you not all over her like a damned rash?"

"Aren't you supposed to be warning me off women?"

Tate blanched. "Why the hell would I do that?"

Max shrugged. "The whole relationships aren't a good idea during recovery spiel?"

Tate gave an innocuous blink. "Well, yeah, but who the hell's talking about a relationship?"

Max snorted and ran a hand through his hair. "We're friends."

"With benefits?"

Max stared at his cup. "Sort of."

Tate sat back, grabbed his cane at his side, and took a deep breath. "We need more coffee and one of those fucking muffins"—he stood—"and then *you* are gonna tell me everything."

It was going to be a long-ass morning.

•   •   •

At three thirty, Max arrived at the cottage. It was a gorgeous day. The sky was clear and the smell of the upcoming summer wafted on the hazy breeze. Grace stood by the stream, her camera to her face as it always was, while she took pictures of the water. She was dressed in a denim skirt, which landed midthigh, a white vest, which made her skin appear lusciously darker, and flip-flops. She'd fastened the top of her hair so the rest fell down her back in jet-black waves and curls. She looked understatedly sexy.

Max made sure he made enough noise to alert her to his presence. She looked up and smiled wide and undisputedly happy. Tate's words echoed in Max's head. Was she hot for him? There was most definitely a mutual attraction. She wouldn't have asked him to sleep with her if there wasn't, right? He pulled his shades off and gave himself a mental slap. He needed to chill the fuck out. Enough with the overthinking.

"You're here," she said.

He opened his arms wide. "Said I would be."

She made an eek face. "You might not be when I tell you why you're here."

Max frowned. "Hit me."

She fisted her hands together, her fingers turning to knots. "So last week when I saw my brother, he told me that I've been commissioned for an art and photography exhibition at the end of August."

Max grinned. "That's amazing."

Grace flushed. "Yeah, it is. It's the first since . . . well, everything, and I'm nervous as hell. My brother's pulled various strings with some friends, but it's great. It's a lot of space to fill, but I won't let that worry me."

"So what do you need me for?"

She took a deep breath. "I was wondering if you'd let me take some pictures of you." Max opened his mouth to protest with a huge, fat "fuck no" but Grace beat him to it. "They're not portraits or anything," she assured him. "In fact, people won't even know it's you. It'll be parts of you."

Max's hands found his hips. "*Parts* of me."

"Mmhm. Like your arms." She lifted her hand but kept it from touching him. "Your chest." The nervous demeanor he'd seen in the coffee shop returned, her expression wary, guarded.

She'd never been that way with Max and he wasn't about to let her start. Without thought, he took a step forward. Grace's hand splayed against his chest, directly above his heart. Her palm burned hot through his tee. A small gasp escaped her at the same time her large eyes snapped to his, all emerald shine and beautiful.

"You can touch me," Max told her gently. "Don't be afraid. Not of me."

She swallowed but didn't move away. Instead, she opened her fingers wider and pressed her palm more firmly against him. An expression of determination hardened her features.

"All right," she whispered. "I'd also want pictures of your face." She lifted her hand gradually, took his chin between her thumb and forefinger, and turned his head to the side. "This part." She traced an invisible line from the corner of his eye to the edge of his mouth with the tip of her finger. "No one would know it's you."

Max's breathing was heavier; his pulse thundered. The feel of Grace's fingers on his jaw, the sensation of her skin against his was unbelievable. It'd been too damned long since he'd experienced a woman's touch. He was hard and breathless and they were both still fully clothed.

Fuck.

"Okay," he croaked.

"Okay?" she asked, dropping her hand. "You'll do it?"

Right then, he'd have done anything she damn well wanted if she'd simply touch him again. "Sure."

For the next hour, Grace took photographs of Max's face, his eyes, his mouth, and his jaw, set against the backdrop of the old cottage, the trees, and the water. She showed him what she'd taken after each one, reassuring him that he was unidentifiable. Max had to admit, though with little surprise, that she was very talented. Her eye for shape and light was extraordinary.

"I need you over there," she ordered, pointing to the over-turned tree he sat on when they had a break on their morning run. He threw one leg over the side, straddling it. Grace sat down next to him.

"I want to take photographs of your hands." Her voice quieted when she touched the back of his wrist. "But, I . . . I want to show color variation." She put her hand on his. "Like this."

Max licked his lips as he looked at their hands together, her skin an exquisite dark, warm caramel against his white and slightly tanned. She lifted her camera with her free hand and clicked twice. She adjusted herself, moving closer, the scent of her perfume, all sweet and floral, accosting Max. She tilted and clicked, moved her hand, moved his, but still she seemed unsatisfied. Max, however, was anything but.

Grace huffed and sat back, removing her fingers from his. "It's not working." She closed her eyes and tilted her head back. "I can't get the angle right."

Max's gaze wandered the length of her neck, across her pulse points, down to the V of her top and the swell of her chest, to the top of her thighs, where her skirt had ridden up. Her legs were fucking perfection. She had runner's legs, slender and strong. He wondered fleetingly what they'd feel like wrapped around his hips, his ribs, and his neck. He bet she tasted incredible.

"You need both hands to hold the camera," he suggested, his voice deep and husky, his stare unmoving from her lap.

"Yeah, but I can't do that while we're"—she gestured between them, frustrated—"sitting like this."

Max took her hand and held it between his, determined. He waited for her to look at him, which she did, blatantly surprised by his directness. But Max was tired of dancing around the issue. If she wanted him to help her, it was time to prove it.

"Do you trust me?" he asked quietly.

Her gaze flickered across him, from his eyes to his mouth, to his hands and back again. Max liked the way her eyes felt on him, innocent and honest. She was silent for an age, causing sweat to gather at his hairline. "Do you?"

She nodded, her stare never wavering. "Yes," she replied. "I trust you."

Max exhaled. "Good." He smiled. "I think I know how we can make this easier." She waited. "Turn around," he said. "So your back's to my chest."

She paused for a moment, took a deep breath, and turned as he asked. She sat back gradually between Max's legs, shuffling across the log until her hair was under his nose, smelling all sorts of awesome, like clean laundry and honey. He needed to know what skin lotion she used, too, because that shit was golden. Nothing could beat the smell of a woman and dammit he'd missed it.

"Place your feet on the tree," he instructed. "Good. Now, I'm gonna place my hands on your legs, okay? That way you can hold the camera and take the picture."

She cleared her throat, but didn't answer. Max sat forward, placing his chin on her shoulder, keeping his hands to himself. "If you don't want to, it's all right," he whispered. "I won't do anything you don't want me to. I swear." She nodded. "Talk to me," he urged. "Tell me what you can handle."

She was breathing quicker. "I'm . . . it's fine." She pursed her lips. Max recognized the calming technique Elliot had taught him when he first entered rehab. "Just . . . go slow. Please."

"Whatever you need."

Max swallowed, adjusting his position behind her, not wanting Grace to feel his lust poking her in the lower back. Jesus, he was wound tighter than a fucking spring. He was suddenly aware of everything about the woman sitting between his legs, her breathing, her scent, the slight tremor in her spine, and when his palms finally made contact with the skin of her legs, he all but gulped the groan that threatened at the back of his throat. She was warm and so fucking soft under his fingertips.

He kept his hands still, pressing into her thighs, his digits reaching the top of her knee. "Take the picture," he murmured into her hair, desperately ignoring the epic view he had down her bra. "Take it."

"I can't move," she gasped.

"Yes, you can." Max shifted his hands, a whisper of skin against skin. "I'm not holding you down. You're in control. You can move, you can push me awa—"

"No, don't," she interrupted with an abrupt shake of her head. "Don't move away."

Max smiled. "I won't."

He wasn't going anywhere. Dammit, what he would have given to push her legs open and feel what delights she had between them. He wondered if she was wet, if she was bare, or as nature intended. He'd turn her around, sit her on his cock, and fuck her hard enough to make her forget everything and everyone she was afraid of, or better yet, he'd bend her over the very log they were sitting on and make her scream his name.

But he knew it wasn't the time for anything but baby steps.

Gentle, slow baby steps.

Fucking would come later.

He closed his eyes and breathed, calming his body down. It was no easy feat. After a moment's silence, Grace lifted the camera and started clicking, taking picture after picture of his hands on her.

"Can you . . . put your hands closer—here, to the inside of my thighs?" Her voice was shy, warm, and incredibly sensual.

Max did as she asked, biting his lip as a secondary urge to cop a feel crashed over him. "Your skin's so soft," he whispered instead, nuzzling her neck, emboldened and relieved as shit that she wasn't freaking out.

Her head dropped back onto his shoulder after she'd taken more pictures.

"It smells good, too," Max continued, taking a huge whiff. "Fuck, what is that?"

She laughed, the motion of it causing her body to rub Max's in nightmarishly fantastic ways. "It's cocoa butter," she murmured.

"It's fucking awesome." She laughed again. Max bit back a groan. "You smell good enough to eat."

The exhale that left Grace's mouth was hungry and wanton and caused Max's fingers to grip her a little harder.

"You're so hot, Gracie," he told her. "So fucking hot." His tongue was out of his mouth and licking a path up her neck before he could comprehend the desire to do it.

"Oh, God," she gasped, leaning her head to the side to give him more access.

Keeping his mouth at her jawline, Max risked moving his hands again, farther between her thighs. His fingers spread so that his thumbs disappeared under her skirt. "I can't wait to feel you," he said against her earlobe. "Here." His hands moved again, teasing, mere inches from where he was desperate to touch. "I'll make it so good, Grace. You have no fucking idea."

Her fingers pushed into the gaps in between his. "I know you will."

Just as Max started to ponder what she'd do if he touched her tits, Grace began to fidget. Max held back a grumble when she gradually moved his palms away. He couldn't complain. She'd allowed him to do so much more than he imagined, and considering the things he knew about what she'd been through, he had to concede that they'd made massive progress. She sat forward and turned to him, her feet resting back on the ground.

Her gaze flitted to his crotch and the tent he was pitching in his cargo shorts. She hid her knowing but embarrassed smile with the back of her hand.

Max chuckled. "I'm not going to apologize about you making me hard," he stated as he stood and stretched with a groan, needing to go for a run to burn off his horniness.

"I wouldn't want you to. I like it."

Max cocked an eyebrow. Her flirty tone was not conducive to getting rid of a righteous boner. "Yeah?"

She shrugged. "Of course. It makes me feel good that you find me attractive."

Max snorted. "Duh."

Grace didn't laugh as Max expected. Instead, she wrapped her arms around herself, making her body smaller. Her eyes cast down.

Max frowned. Panic teased his neck. "I didn't mean to freak you out. You should have told me if I did too much. Did I do too much?"

"No!" she all but shouted. "No. Max, it was . . . I—I liked it. Very much. You did nothing wrong."

He approached slowly, sitting at her side. "Then what is it?" She bit her lip and sighed. Max moved her hair from her shoulder down her back. "Grace, tell me."

"I want to give back," she whispered, glancing at his lap. "I want to touch you, too."

"You can," he insisted. Was she crazy? "Look, like I said, I'm a guy, so you want to touch me? Touch me. Shit, girl, you wanna hump me in public? You hump me in public. You want to put your hands in my pants? Put your damned hands in my pants."

She laughed then, making Max smile. "I'm not sure we're at the humping-in-public stage quite yet."

"Ha!" Max pointed a finger at her. "That wasn't a no! Does that mean you would?"

She pushed him playfully. "Shut up! Perv."

The warm breeze whipped around them, making the leaves of the trees rustle.

"Don't be scared of using me," Max added seriously. He continued before she could object to his word choice. "Use me to find out what you want, what your boundaries are, what makes you feel good. That's what we're doing here, right?"

She observed him for a moment, her stare intense. "Okay." She leaned over and kissed his cheek quickly. "Thank you."

17

Grace took photographs of Max almost every day.

When they were running, when they were hanging out, when he was working at the house. Okay, if Grace was truly honest, most of the photographs she took were done so covertly and were for her own private collection rather than for the show.

Max simply had the most exquisite and photogenic face. If she didn't like him so much, she'd have hated him for it.

He was all hard edges, scars—he had two, one on his right eyebrow and one on his chin—and masculine lines. His hair was so dark it was almost black, as were his eyes, but when the sun caught the shadowy scruff on his face, it shone bright gold and auburn, while his eyes flickered with hazel and chocolate. He truly was beautiful.

And apparently had the patience of a saint.

The two of them hadn't touched the way they had since their day by the cottage, a day that Grace had thought about constantly. There'd been hand brushes and shoulder nudges, but nothing that had set her alight as much as his hands on her thighs had done. Sweet Jesus, Grace was amazed that she hadn't burst into actual flames. It'd been the first time in too long that she hadn't shied away from a man's touch.

And what a touch it was.

The rough, callused skin and the long, firm fingers of his hands could have brought her to orgasm without him going anywhere near her panties. It was gentle but commanding and even after she'd moved his hands away, she still felt them on her thighs a week later.

As surprised as she'd been that Max had taken the initiative and touched her, Grace was even more surprised at herself. Of course, there had been initial panic that squeezed her lungs and made her heart pump, but the peak of it was over as quickly as it had begun. By the time Max's tongue was making its way up her neck and he was whispering devilish words into her ear, Grace's heart was crashing behind her ribs for an altogether different reason.

She was aroused.

Like, truly, achingly turned on for the first time in years.

Max's touch, his body pressed into hers along with his sexy mutterings, had awoken her libido with a giant how *you* doin'? Her blood heated, her breathing grew labored, and Grace knew that if she hadn't pulled his hands away, they'd have gone a lot further.

But it would have been too fast. She had to remember to take it all one step at a time. For as proud of herself as Grace was, there were still elements of intimacy that scared her to death. She'd tried working them out with her therapist, Nina, over the years, but still the thought of touching a man below the hips left her more than a little apprehensive. Nina had urged her to take a chance when Grace had mentioned her deal with Max. Let go, she'd said; don't be afraid of pleasure.

And she didn't want to be. Seeing Max so hard for her was as exciting as it was nerve-racking. She wanted to touch him. Almost desperately, just to see what he felt like, to see if she could make him come, but every time she thought about doing it, uneasiness ravaged her.

"Hey, Grace?"

Grace turned from adjusting the cushions on her new leather sofa to see Buck and another of Vince's workers staggering into the front door with a huge box between them. From the bend of their legs, it was very heavy.

"Vanity desk in the bedroom?" Buck gasped.

God bless him. He'd done nothing but apologize to Grace after his birthday and her completely embarrassing freak-out. He'd even bought her flowers. Daisies. He couldn't do enough. His affection had certainly endeared him to her.

"Please," Grace answered. "Thank you!" She smiled when the two men heaved and groaned as they started their journey up the stairway.

The house was finally completed. Grace glanced around, the smile on her face enormous. She'd done it. She finally owned something that was hers, untainted by her past, something that she'd done on her own. It was so beautiful and homey and exactly what Grace had dreamed about. She'd done nothing but dash around it, holding in her girlie squeals of excitement at the wooden floors, high ceilings, and wide windows. She couldn't wait for Kai to see it. It even had a blue door. It was perfect.

Most of her furniture had arrived over two days, all except her bed, though the blowup mattress Ruby had loaned her was just fine for the time being. Vince had offered the moving services of his workers and anyone else who'd been in the bar the night they celebrated the house's completion. Even Ruby had offered her husband's muscles, as well as her own sandwich- and lemonade-making skills, which came in handy when the workers started wilting in the heat. It was a comforting feeling having such amazing people around her.

Max missed the celebration, being away at one of his meetings, but he'd helped the day after, moving wardrobes, sofas, and fridge freezers. Grace would catch his eyes on her repeatedly. She'd smile and he'd smile back, subtle and cool, but still it made her stomach dance.

When the last of the helpers left, each with a pack of beer, which Grace had bought as thanks, she made her way to the boardinghouse to see Max. She knocked on his room door as best as she could with her hands full. When she heard him call out, she did her best to disregard the fluttering in her belly. And when she heard his footsteps approach, she grinned when he opened the door, but it dropped off her face like a lead weight.

Holy. Shit.

If Grace had found Max attractive with his clothes on, it was a whoooole other story seeing him without. He was bare-chested and barefoot, wearing only a loose pair of black sweats, which sat low on his hips and were splattered with various colors of paint. The V of his torso was defined enough to have every pair of panties in a ten mile radius combusting at a geometric rate. His stomach was flat with grooves of muscle and a smattering of dark hair that trailed down from his broad chest. His shoulders were thick and strong.

And, oh my God, was that a *tattoo*—

"It's rude to stare."

Grace's eyes snapped to Max's face. Arrogant bastard was smirking, leaning a forearm on the doorjamb, twiddling a paint-brush between his fingers. He even had the audacity to waggle his eyebrows.

"I wasn't staring," she lied. She cleared her throat and shook her head in an attempt to clear the foggy lust suddenly smother-ing her brain. "I wouldn't. I was simply . . . you know, I was just looking at— Look, I brought pizza." She lifted the large box in one hand. "Pepperoni, with extra onion. And Dr Pepper." She lifted the other.

"Well, then you'd better come in," he said with a laugh, prop-ping the door open for her.

Grace entered, dipping beneath his arm, her cheeks flaming hot under his knowing gaze.

His room was set out exactly as hers had been, except there were a set of heavy-looking dumbbells in the corner and a large canvas set up on a tripod, surrounded by an array of paints and brushes. A large sheet hid the picture, and Grace's fingers itched to lift it up and peek at his work. Several other canvases, turned from view, leaned against the far wall.

"You've been painting?" she asked, placing the pizza and soda on a small side table. "Is that why I haven't seen you?"

Max rubbed a hand across his stomach, watching her every move. "I've done a little. Nothing exciting." He moved toward her, putting his paintbrush down, and lifted the pizza box lid. "I'm starving." The bite he took of the slice he picked up was gargantuan.

Grace tried hard not to watch his jaw work and his neck move with his swallow. She tried *really* hard. She shifted toward the paintings, her finger dancing over the top of them. "Do you ever let anyone see your work?" she asked nonchalantly.

Max shrugged, picking up a second piece of pizza. "Sometimes." He watched her a moment before rolling his eyes. "You can look if you want. It's not a national secret or anything."

Grace beamed at him before she began turning the canvases around. Each one was very different, but every one affirmed what Grace already knew: Max was seriously talented. The colors and shades that he used were bold and aggressive in some, while others were more subtle, careful, calmer. The asymmetric shapes and patterns he used drew the eye over every inch of the painting, whispering in light greens, soft browns, and silent black and screaming with blood red. His voice was blatant in each one, angry in some, smart and sensitive in others. As Grace regarded each one carefully, she noticed how the ire became less and less obvious in each one; the shapes became less harsh, less angular, and more sweeping, curved, and gentle. She smiled.

"They're amazing, Max," she told him, standing from her crouched position. "Really. You're very good." Her finger traced the subtle pink splashes of the one closest to her, her favorite. "They should be shown off somewhere."

Max snorted and shook his head. "No one wants them. I couldn't even give them away."

"I'd have them," she retorted quickly. "This one, at least. I love it." The sweeping caramels and hints of gold reminded Grace of her mother's eyes.

Max waved a hand, not really paying attention. "Then it's yours." He grabbed another slice of pizza. "This is epic. What did I do to deserve all this?"

Grace didn't comment on the sharp deviation in conversation as she approached him. She knew that he'd probably allowed her to say and do much more than he would ordinarily, and she appreciated that. Max was a private person and, as a fellow artist, Grace understood how personal one's work was.

"It's just a small thank-you for all your help with the house," she replied. "I gave the rest of the guys beer, but I thought you'd appreciate this more." She ventured to the bathroom to grab some toilet paper to use as makeshift napkins.

"You were right." Max dropped down onto the side of the bed after swiping a can of Dr Pepper. "I love pizza."

Grace snorted and joined him with her own slice and a can, hyperaware that he'd still not put on a shirt and they were sitting on his sheet-rumpled bed. Under the delicious aroma of oregano and pepperoni floating around them, the underlying scent of man enveloped her. Her pulse jumped but, weirdly, panic never took hold.

"So how did this morning go?"

Max had had an appointment with his therapist, causing him to miss their run. She didn't mind, obviously, but his absence did make the day drag a little bit longer, even with all the chaos at the house.

"Good," Max said after swallowing a bite of pizza. "He's lowered my meds. Says he's pleased with my progress."

"That's great," Grace enthused. "I'm proud of you."

Max looked at her dubiously, wiping his mouth. "You are?"

"Sure." She shrugged. "It's great that you're doing so well."

"Like you." He nudged her elbow with his own. "You must be stoked that the house is done."

"Yeah. Although I'll miss not having you across the hall."

He chuckled. "Well, you know who to call if your pipes fuck up."

Grace swallowed the last of her pizza as well as the nerves festering in her throat. "You're more than welcome to come over," she murmured. She fiddled with her soda can. "Whenever you want. Anytime. I could cook for you."

She chanced a glance at Max. He appeared amused, his lips twitching as though fighting a grin. "Sure, I'll come over. Especially if you're cooking. Man's gotta eat, right?" He shoveled another slice of pizza into his mouth.

As he lifted his arm, Grace noticed a large scar that ran from under his left pec, horizontally across his ribs, toward his back. Her fingers reached out to touch it before she could stop herself. Not that Max appeared to mind. He looked down at where her fingers traced the deep groove of healed flesh.

"Ah. That," he mumbled around his food.

"What did this?" she asked quietly.

"A bullet."

Max's answer was so matter-of-fact that it took Grace a moment to comprehend what he'd said. When the words settled in her brain, she startled, yanking her hand away. "A bull— Are you serious?"

He nodded, still chewing.

"What happened?"

"My best friend and I got caught up in some shit."

"Carter?" Max spoke about his friend often. He clearly cared for him, talking of him as more like a brother than a friend.

"Yeah." He placed his hand on the scar. "This was from a car boost that went wrong."

Grace sat back, bewilderment prickling her skin. "You're so cavalier about it."

"I don't mean to be. It is what it is and it happened a long time ago."

"Did it do any damage?"

"Only what you can see. I was lucky. The doc said because of how I pushed Carter out of the way, the bullet missed its true trajectory." He patted his chest. "My heart."

Grace frowned. "Wait. You pushed Carter out of the way?"

"Yeah. The fucker with his finger on the trigger aimed at my boy from across the street."

"Jesus." Grace crossed her arms over herself, suddenly cold despite the humidity of the room. "You could have been killed."

Max shrugged. "He's my best friend. No one's allowed to shoot him but me." He smiled toward the floor.

The plot surrounding Max O'Hare thickened. Bullets, car boosting, and drugs. *Oh my.* To any normal, *sane* individual, they were all words that should have had Grace bolting for the door, and hightailing it far, far away. Yet the modesty with which he talked about saving his friend's life kept her ass firmly in place. There was so much more to him than swagger and rehab and Grace couldn't deny the hunger to learn it all. The paintings were a mere glimpse into what made him tick.

Max placed his can on the floor and turned toward her, resting his palm on the bed. "I'm not proud of my past, as you well know, but I can't change it. This scar is just one of the things in my life that remind me of who I don't want to be."

"And your tattoo?" she asked, gesturing to the curve of black ink that swept across his shoulder and the upper bicep of his right arm. Grace wanted him to turn around so she could see the rest of it.

He smiled wryly, shaking his head. "That's a story for another day, I think."

Disappointed, she nodded in acquiescence.

Grace could understand his point about trying to get away from the past, however. The scars on the skin of her ribs and hip were an ugly reminder of what she'd never allow herself to go through again. Wanting to share, she shifted from her place on the bed's edge, turned, and slowly lifted her T-shirt.

For a moment, Max appeared puzzled, before his stare landed on the pale scars running in zigzags from underneath her right breast to her hip. Max inhaled deeply, his jaw twitching.

"What did this?" he asked, repeating her question, even though the tone of his voice suggested he knew.

"A size-eleven foot and a kitchen knife."

The deep rumble that emitted from Max's throat sounded like a growl. "Motherfucker." He exhaled and reached out his hand. "Can I?"

Grace blinked in reply. His large fingers whispered across her scars as if she were made of glass.

"They're ugly, huh?" She tried to smile around the words, closing her eyes to the sensation of his touch, the tenderness that he drew on her skin with his fingertips.

"No," Max retorted firmly. "They're not."

"You don't have to lie. It's okay."

Max sighed, dropping his hand from her. "When my dad first got cancer, he had tons of surgeries. He had scars everywhere from the top of his head to his belly. I asked him once if they embarrassed him, if he hated them. He laughed and said, 'How can I hate them? They show everyone what I've survived.'"

He pressed his palm to her side again, its heat soaked deep into Grace's bones. His dark stare pinned her in place. "These scars show everyone what you survived, Grace. Don't you dare be ashamed of them."

Tears pricked Grace's eyes and her breath shuddered out, his words fracturing years of self-conscious anxiety and indignity in mere seconds. He moved his hand, cupping her side, moving down toward her hip. The span of his hand was mammoth against her small waist. He licked his lips, his tongue a gorgeous pink. "You're so soft."

He shifted closer, their knees touched, and his fingers skimmed the underneath of her bra, sending Grace's lungs into a frenzy. "I love your hands on me," she breathed, because it was the truth, because she needed him to know, because she'd die if he took them away.

"Show me more," he murmured, looking at her through his long black lashes. "It's just us. Be brave with me. Let me see you."

Without a moment's hesitation, Grace lifted the hem of her top up and over her head, leaving her in a hot pink bra and yoga pants. Max hummed a deep, sensual sound that curled Grace's toes and reached his hands to her collarbone. She didn't even flinch.

"That's it," he sighed. "Look at you."

His touch was fire and safety and awoke a dormant part of Grace that had her reaching to unfasten the hooks at her back.

Max noticed her movement and huffed out a breath. "Only if you're comfortable."

"I want to let go. I want you to see. I want to be brave," she whispered and unhooked, pulling the cups away from her chest and the straps from her shoulders, so they were both naked from the waist up.

"Sweet Jesus," Max uttered. "You're . . ." His fingers slid across her collarbone and down. His gaze flickered to hers the closer he got to her breasts, caution in their depths. "All right?"

"Yes."

And she was. Oh, God, she was. She felt alive in his hands, and when he finally touched her nipples and cupped her in his palms, she moaned a sound she didn't know she was capable of. It was relief, gratitude, and yearning for more. He groaned, too, as he squeezed her gently, tweaking her nipples between his thumb and forefingers, moving closer.

His tongue poked out between his open lips. "You have such

great tits." His thumb circled her. "Perfect. Look how they fit my hands." He watched, his gaze hot and enraptured as her breasts moved and rippled under his ministrations. "Fuck, Grace, I want— Will you let me, can I suck them?"

His words were so unintentionally erotic, Grace could do nothing but nod.

He leaned closer. "I've got you. You're safe," he murmured. "And so fucking sexy."

And then his mouth was on her.

His burning tongue wound around her nipple, flicking, teasing, and sending electricity coursing through her veins. It was wet, sloppy, and made Grace call out and sag against him. He hummed into her skin, sucking harder, grabbing tighter, breathing harder. Grace's body twitched and grew wet, desperate for friction, but fearful of having his body over hers, holding her down. She pushed her hands into his hair, sighing at its thickness between her fingers, wanting nothing more than to bury her nose into it and breathe him in. She held him close.

She was safe, she reminded herself. He wasn't going to hurt her.

"Feels so good," she murmured, knowing from the ache between her legs that she could easily come from his mouth on her chest alone.

Max's reply was muffled but loud and, when Grace looked, she saw that he was rubbing himself furiously through his sweats with the heel of his hand.

"Oh, God," she gasped, yearning flashing through her. "Please let me see."

His mouth never moved, but his eyes darkened impossibly further as they flickered up.

"Could you come?" she asked. He nodded, his lips sliding against her. "Show me."

He pulled down his waistband and underwear faster than Grace could take another breath. The head of his cock slapped his belly, glistening and so very hard. No cock she'd ever seen was pretty, but Grace would say that Max's was magnificent. He was thick and long and when he twisted his fist over its bulbous tip, Max moaned and sucked her harder. That was good to know for when she touched him there.

And she *would* touch him there.

There was no question.

Desire curled in her belly, tighter and tighter as images of them doing more, going further, pummeled her mind until she, too, was pushing her hand into her pants and into her underwear. She was drenched and burning. One swipe of the pad of her thumb against her clit and her back arched. Her head hit the headboard and she cried out.

Max released her nipple with a loud smack of his lips, his eyes widening when he saw what she was doing. "Fuck, are you touching yourself?"

She bit her lip and nodded—his words gasoline to an already furious inferno. "Close."

Even though her eyes were closed, Grace knew Max's fist had sped up. The bed shook and his grunts got louder, his breath hot and wild on her throat.

"Are you imagining it?" he asked. His voice was wicked, dark, and hungry. "Are you imagining what my fingers would feel like on you, in you? What my cock would feel like as you rode it?"

So close.

So near to falling.

"Yeah, you are. I know you are. You know I'd fuck you so good." He licked her jaw. "Right after I'd devoured you down there, I'd slide right in and have you screaming my name." He heaved a breath. "I'd do anything you damn well wanted me to, woman. Anywhere. *Shit.* Fuck, Gracie, can I come on you?"

And those were all the words she needed to explode into a thousand pieces.

As her back bowed and white-hot ecstasy all but sliced her in two, Grace was aware of warmth splashing up the middle of her torso, while Max's guttural groans were enough to keep her orgasm rolling incessantly through every inch of her body. She wished she'd been able to see him come, but her eyes were forced shut by the pleasure vibrating her very bones, bright lights filling her vision. She pulsed and gasped while Max's voice became gruff and breathless in her ear.

"I've got you, Gracie," he husked. "You're okay. I've got you."

As she calmed and her body returned to the earth, his hands and face gradually moved away. "Fuck," Max bit out after a moment where their heavy breathing was all that could be heard. "Christ, I needed that."

Grace regained the use of her eyes just as Max dropped back onto the bed, making it bounce. His pants were back in place; while his arms spread wide, a small smile played on his face and he closed his eyes. The faint gleam of sweat across his chest looked good enough to lick. She imagined he tasted exquisite. Glancing down, Grace saw the remnants of Max's orgasm, white and stretching from her belly button to her collarbone. Grace couldn't remember seeing something so sensual, something that should have been dirty and gross, but just . . . wasn't.

If anything, it was the most beautiful thing she'd ever seen. It was freedom and hope. It represented what she'd overcome. It represented what she made Max feel, what she could do for him, what she was capable of doing to a man, this man, and for the first time in years, Grace's confidence stood up a little straighter. She didn't even feel the need to cover up her naked chest.

"Are you okay?"

Grace looked over at Max. His brow furrowed gently when he noticed where her attention was.

"Was it all right that I did that?" he asked, sitting up and reaching for some of the leftover toilet paper.

"It was . . ." Grace took the paper he held out to her but made no attempt to move or wipe Max off her skin. She stared at him. "It was hot as fuck."

Max's laugh exploded out of him, making his face crinkle and his shoulders shake. "One orgasm and she's got a mouth on her like a sailor." He shook his head and rubbed his hands through his hair, making it stand up in a million and one different directions. "Well, hell, we might just have to try that shit again sometime."

Grace grinned.

You bet your ass we will.

18

"So, do you have plans for July Fourth?"

Grace looked over at Ruby, who was running at her side. She was red in the cheeks and breathing hard, but she kept up with Grace, stride for stride, despite the two of them being running buddies for a grand total of four days.

From the ass crack of dawn until late every night, Max had been working with his uncle Vince out of town and, as a result, was too tired to do anything, least of all run. It wasn't good news for Grace's libido, but she tried to be understanding. Ruby had eagerly stepped in as Grace's partner, citing the need to get rid of her muffin top and get ready for new bikinis. Grace couldn't see even a hint of a muffin top on Ruby's petite frame, but kept quiet. Ruby had always been nice to her, with the added extra of being really fun to be around.

"July Fourth? Not that I'm aware of."

"Great! Wanna come to my dad's cabin for a few days? There's a group of us goin'. We do it every year. It's by the lake so you can swim every day, we go out on the boat, we grill, cook s'mores, get drunk, fool around, plus the fireworks are incredible. It's good fun."

It sure did sound it; still, caution itched at Grace's neck. She wasn't working and she'd made no plans with Kai, knowing that he'd be jetting off somewhere with his new set of boobs or his buddies. "Um, I don't know."

"Oh, come on!" Ruby encouraged. "It'll be fantastic. You'll

know most of the people there." She started lifting fingers with each name. "Me, Josh, Dad and Mom, obviously, Caleb, Buck and a couple of his lady friends, and Max."

That piqued her interest. Grace slowed to a walk, placing her hands on her hips. "Max is going?" She tried to hide the obvious curiosity in her voice, but from the glint in Ruby's eye, she'd failed miserably.

"Mmhm," Ruby replied with a smirk, still jogging on the spot. The cute, pink, bow-shaped clips she had in her hair to keep her short bangs back bounced as she did. "What's going on with you two anyhow?"

Grace shook her head, the image of his orgasm all over her still fresh and still sexy as all get-out. "Nothing's going on. We're friends."

Ruby's mile widened. "You like him, don't you?"

Grace cleared her throat and avoided Ruby's smiling eyes by pretending to stretch. "Who are we talking about?"

Ruby snorted. "My cousin. Max. You know, the guy you're always with, the guy you can't stop looking at, the guy who lights up every time you walk into the room."

Grace's head snapped up. "He does not."

"Ah!" Ruby retorted with a grin and a pointing finger. "But you'd like him to."

Grace exhaled, not knowing whether to be relieved or hurt that Ruby was playing with her. She rubbed a palm down her face and kicked at a nearby stone, confusion drying her throat. Over the weeks, and with all the time she'd spent with him, it had slowly become apparent that her investment in the agreement she had with Max was tilting toward something less friends-only and more dangerous, something scary and new.

"Yeah," she murmured toward the ground. "I like him." The confession should have been freeing—it was the truth, after all— yet the words made Grace hollow. She looked up.

Ruby was standing closer, no longer moving. She smiled gently. "Max is a decent guy. He's messed up, which isn't surprising given what he's been through, but he has a good heart."

Grace nodded in agreement. "He does."

Ruby crossed her arms. "You could be good for him."

"I don't know." Grace sighed.

He'd told her, in no uncertain terms, that he couldn't give her anything but his body. A few weeks ago, Grace had been fine with that—and she still was. Sometimes. Other times, when his hands were on her . . . She gave her head a shake and breathed. She knew she was being ridiculous. It wasn't anything other than excitement she was feeling. Excitement about the progress she was making with intimacy, at the leaps she'd made being with a man. Besides, she knew, deep down, she wasn't ready for anything serious, either. It was just . . . Max made her *feel* ready.

"Look, come to the cabin," Ruby said quietly. "See what happens. Max is always chill when he's at the lake. You two can maybe have some *fun*." She cocked an eyebrow. "If you get my meaning."

Grace laughed, shielding her heated cheeks with her hands. Yeah, she got Ruby's meaning and, she had to admit, if going to the cabin meant she and Max could be alone to have some more "fun," then she was all for it. She could brush aside her confusion and treacherous emotions for now.

Hiding her feelings, good or bad, was not a new thing for her or her heart.

• • •

The drive up to the cabin was as long and hot as it always was. Max was grateful he wasn't the one behind the wheel for once. He was sitting in the back of his uncle's pickup, alongside Ruby and Josh, admiring the views and looking forward to a few days of rest and relaxation. He couldn't wait to get in the lake. It was amazing this time of year, and the treks into the mountains were great for walks or runs. He'd have to show Grace. She'd appreciate it for the photography potential.

When Max had learned that Grace would be joining them all at the cabin, he'd been pleased. He was genuinely happy that she'd made friends with Ruby and that everyone had welcomed her so thoroughly. But that was just his family. They were cool like that. He liked that they liked her and that she was becoming less and less timid, becoming braver, more inclined to take on new challenges. He was proud of her when he heard her sass the way she did when it was just the two of them.

He just didn't like it when she did it with Deputy Asswipe.

Max hadn't peeked at the truck following theirs. He'd managed to ignore the urge for at least thirty minutes already and he wasn't backing down now. Nope. He didn't give a flying shit that Grace was in Deputy Asshole's ride with Buck and two random women. Not at all.

He fidgeted, checking his cell. No signal. Damn mountains.

He glanced back.

Buck waved back wildly between the front seats, nudging Grace, who laughed and waved, too.

Fucker.

Max noted the deputy's sly expression and clenched his fist. He understood that Uncle Vince had known the deputy for a long time, but did the prick really have to join them at the lake? The answer was apparently yes, since, as Ruby explained, he'd been doing so for the past four summers. Whatever. Max only just managed to resist the urge to flip the bird or write out a text message to show the jerk later, describing in detail how Grace's tits tasted and felt on his tongue, or what his orgasm looked like all over her skin, or the smell of her body after she'd come. But that might have been a tad overzealous.

Nevertheless, those particular images had entertained Max and his cock no end for days. Dammit, he couldn't wait to get Grace alone again, so he could see what else she had lurking under that innocent quiet of hers. The tigress he'd glimpsed was ridiculously hot, and Max knew that once he got the chance to tear away the rest of her apprehension, she'd be unstoppable.

The man she'd end up with would certainly have a tomcat on his hands. He just hoped to God that it wasn't Deputy AssBandit. For whatever reason, the dude rubbed Max the wrong way and how he looked at Grace, as if she were a piece of meat or something, made Max's teeth grind. He wasn't good enough for her and Max was more than prepared to set that shit straight anytime the prick wanted.

Thirty minutes later, with a barrage of hootin' and hollerin' from the truck's occupants, Max's uncle pulled up outside the cabin. The place hadn't changed one bit since Max's last visit, twelve years before. Predominantly logged, with a few modern metal and glass embellishments that Uncle Vince added over the years, the six-bedroom cabin sat one hundred feet back from the water, a gorgeous lake three miles long and one mile wide. Max had spent many a summer swimming, fishing, and boating on that lake with his uncle and his father, and as he stepped out of the truck and took in the beauty of it, nostalgia trembled through him. The memories he had at the cabin were happy ones, trouble-free ones, ones that every kid should have.

"Penny for them."

Max startled at the sound of Grace's voice. She was standing at his side in a pair of denim shorts, a pink tank top, and matching flip-flops. As always, her toes were painted the exact same color as her outfit.

"Nice ride up?" He cocked an eyebrow over his shades.

She shrugged. "Buck was entertaining as hell. Caleb wouldn't let us put music on. Good music, at least. His tastes leave a lot to be desired."

"Color me shocked as hell," he muttered sarcastically, causing Grace to snort. She lifted her hand to shield her eyes from the glare off the water.

"My goodness it's beautiful here." She breathed in deeply. "I can see why you like it."

Max peered over at her. Her eyes closed as she tilted her face up to the sun. She'd put her hair up into a messy bun that was unable to hold a handful of curling tendrils that hung from it. His eyes roamed over her shoulders and throat.

"Yeah," Max murmured. "Beautiful."

"Guys, come on!" Ruby yelled from behind them, making them both turn. "Get your bags and get changed. Dad's gonna start the grill while we have a swim."

"Best do as she says," Grace said out of the corner of her mouth. "She can be scary."

Max snickered and watched her bound back over to the deputy's truck. Back at his uncle's truck, Max yanked his own bag from its bed and slung it over his shoulder. "Which room am I in?"

Ruby paused and chewed on her lower lip. Max tilted his head. He knew that fucking look from when they were kids. "What did you do?"

"Well," she answered, elongating the vowel. "Buck's friends won't share a room, so we're one short. You'll be okay to share, right?"

He pulled his shades down his nose so he could glare at her better. "With whom?"

Ruby grinned. "Your buddy."

Max's brows snapped together in confusion. "My what?"

"Hey, Grace!" Ruby called out, the volume of her voice belying her tiny stature. "You don't mind bunking in with Max, do you?"

Max turned to see Grace shake her head and quickly drop her eyes to the ground. Max spun back to his cousin, opening his mouth to unleash a barrage of what-the-fuck?

Ruby held up a hand. "Oh, stop," she said with a roll of her eyes. "You're such a drama llama!"

"A drama llama?" Max spluttered incredulously. "Are you fucking high?"

Ruby laughed and shook her head. "Look, it's simple. Grace can either share with you or with Caleb."

"Fuck that," he hissed.

"As I thought," she replied with a knowing smile. "So chill your bean, dude. It's just a hot woman in your room, is all. Relax." Ruby slapped his belly and hurried up to the house.

Max exhaled and stretched his neck, making it crack.

Well, this was sure to make shit interesting.

·   ·   ·

Max opened the bedroom door and threw his bag down at the foot of the bed. The huge bed. The only bed in the entire fucking room. He put his hands on his hips while he watched Grace place her bag next to his. She pressed her lips together and pinched her shoulders, looking small and maddeningly nervous.

"Listen," Max started with a wave of his hand toward the room. It was at the front of the house with picture-perfect views across the water and up the mountains, which could be accessed through French windows that opened onto a private balcony. "Don't worry about all of this. I'll get some blankets and sleep on the floor."

"You will not!" Grace retorted firmly. "This is your break, too." She cleared her throat and glanced at the bed, then back at Max. "I trust you. It'll be fine." She fingered the duvet cover. "Sort of like friends having a sleepover."

Max stared at her for a moment before bursting out laughing. "Sure, a sleepover, but don't for one minute think I'm having pillow fights with you in my underwear."

She didn't miss a beat. "Oh, my friends and I don't bother wearing underwear during *our* pillow fights."

Max's crotch tightened at the same time the breath left his lungs. Holy fuck. She blinked all innocent and shit, waiting for an answer. "Don't tease," he grumbled with a small smirk. "It's not nice."

She laughed and pulled a smaller bag from the depths of the larger. "Who's teasing?" she asked as she walked into the bathroom.

Max rubbed his face. Fucking woman was gonna kill him. He followed her to the bathroom and leaned against the jamb. He watched her place all manner of lotions and potions onto the shelves and around the sink. It was no wonder her skin was as soft and unblemished as it was. Plus it always smelled incredible. His eyes lingered on the back of her thighs and over her ass. He really liked her ass. He wondered whether it was as soft as the rest of her.

"You okay?"

Max blinked, her voice coaxing him from his visual appraisal. She eyed him provocatively in the mirror.

"Yeah," he answered, his voice rough.

"You know," she said, turning slowly and leaning against the sink, "I like it when you look at me like that."

Max swallowed. "Like what?"

"Like that." She nodded toward him. "Like you want me."

He took a step forward, propelled by her large eyes and the rise and fall of her chest. The bathroom filled quickly with heavy anticipation. "I do want you," he answered because why the fuck lie about it? He was aching to touch her, to feel her nipples against his tongue again.

"Good," she replied, lifting her chin to look at him better. "I want you, too."

Max's cock hardened further. He reached out a finger and let the back of it trace the apple of her cheek. Her eyes fluttered closed at the same time her tongue wet her lips. She had a great mouth.

Max had imagined many times what it would look like around him, sucking and kissing where he wanted her most.

"This is all on your terms," he whispered. "You're in control. You just say the word and I'll do whatever the fuck you want me to." His finger moved to her jaw, down her neck, and between her tits. "I want to make you feel good."

"You do," she sighed, reaching for his belt loops and pulling him closer. She looked up. "I want to do the same."

He took her wrist gently and pushed her hand against his cock, grunting softly at the pressure. "I've told you. It's yours to do what you will." His breath made the hair at her temple move.

For one astonishing moment, Max could have sworn her fingers twitched against him, a brief second where he truly thought she was going to take control and touch him properly, but the desire in her pupils steadily fizzled and died, leaving nothing but uncertainty. Trying hard not to take the rejection too personally, Max cleared his throat, released her hand, and stepped back, giving her space.

"I'm sorry," she whispered, staring at the tiled floor beneath their feet.

"Hey," he said sharply. "No. Don't do that. You have nothing to apologize for. Got it?"

She nibbled her bottom lip and sighed.

"Grace?" Max pressed. He didn't like that she felt she had to please him. He wasn't that guy. Sure, he'd felt a twinge of frustration when she'd pulled her hand away, but that was just his cock talking. "No pressure, okay? Seriously." He lifted her chin with his index finger, smiling gently when she didn't flinch. She never flinched around him anymore. "Look, forget about it. And try again when you feel ready."

She nodded, her gaze watery. "Okay."

Max rubbed the tops of her arms. "So how about we go for a swim with these nutjobs, huh?"

She crossed her arms over her chest. "Um, you go. I'll just hang here for a while."

Max bit the inside of his mouth, hating the despondency that cloaked her. He hadn't seen it for weeks and its return was not welcome. "No way, lady; we're here to have fun, not mope. So sort your shit out." He grabbed her forearm and pulled her from the bathroom back into the bedroom. He turned back to her expectantly.

A smile teased at the edges of her lips. "Okay, fine, but I'm not in the mood for swimming. And my new swimsuit doesn't quite cover . . ." She motioned to her side, where Max knew her skin was scarred. His chest squeezed.

"Grace, you know those assholes won't give a shit about that, right?"

"I know," she replied, quickly reaching to play with her hair.

"I don't give a shit about it, either," he added gently, because, if anything, the scars added "fortitude" to the ever-growing list of her endearing traits.

She smiled. "I know, I know. I just . . . Maybe tomorrow. What else can we do?"

Max thought for a moment before an idea pulled his mouth into a wide grin. "You brought your camera?"

"Of course."

"Then let's go."

. . .

For almost two hours, Max showed Grace the nearby treks around the house, leading her through brush, pointing out the breathtaking views of the lake and the surrounding mountains. Grace followed him without question, her trust in him implicit, snapping pictures of the trees, flowers, the exquisite light that filtered through the tree canopy, and a few of Max when he wasn't looking, too involved in describing his adventures in the forests as a kid.

Ruby had been right—Max was a different person at the cabin. He was still the beautiful, gentle man she'd grown to know, but here Grace saw the tension in his shoulders evaporate, while the smile on his face was constantly in place. He was younger, freer, less closed off, and more willing to open up. His stories about his father and their fishing trips were too cute and at times hilarious and had Grace enraptured, especially when, later that evening, seated around a large fire, eating steak and burgers, Vince joined in. Max laughed more than Grace had ever heard, loud and bellied, as memories and anecdotes jumped around the group like a game of hot potato. Grace sat with her glass of wine, listening to the banter, feeling for the first time in years like she was truly at peace. And it was, in no small part, thanks to the man sitting at her side.

"Hey, Max, do you remember the night we snuck into the garage freezer and stole that ice cream we weren't allowed and your dad was convinced there was a bear loose?" Ruby laughed around the rim of her wineglass.

Max snorted and nodded. "Oh my God. We were terrified he was going to find out that we'd stolen it."

Vince shook his head. "You kids were a damned nightmare."

The two "nightmares" fist-bumped. "Solid work, my man." Ruby grinned.

"Word." Max nodded solemnly.

"Why weren't you allowed the ice cream?" Grace asked.

The roars of laughter from Vince, Fern, and Ruby and the blush creeping up Max's cheeks were too intriguing to let go. Grace nudged his shoulder. "What did you do?"

Buck spluttered over his burger. "Man, I heard about this! Was this the naked police incident?"

Whoops of hilarity filled the warm summer evening and drifted along the edge of the water like leaves on a breeze.

"Naked police?" Caleb asked incredulously from his seat next to Vince.

"Damn, boy, I'll never be able to delete those images for as long as I live!" Ruby commented.

Max chuckled into his forearm. "Yeah, right, like you'd want to." He winked and sipped from his bottle of Dr Pepper.

"So, come on," Buck's blonde friend, Carla, said impatiently. "What happened?"

She was pretty, Grace supposed, in a fake-hair-and-boobs, bright-white-teeth kind of way, but the manner in which she'd been eyeing Max all night certainly wasn't.

Max sighed in amusement. "Ruby dared me to flash the family who were staying across the lake." Ruby began to protest over the loud oohs and aahs. "You did," he continued with a pointed finger. "Don't deny it. It was all your fault."

Grace laughed. "And did you?"

"Of course I fucking did. I'd never concede a dare. I couldn't let her win!"

"The only problem was," Ruby sniggered, "as he stood on the float in the middle of the lake and dropped his shorts to greet the poor folks, the local mountain police were doing their morning rounds and saw him!"

Max dropped his head back. "Shit, I was terrified."

"They hauled his ass back to the cabin," Vince added. "He's there standing on the damned porch with only a police hat covering his unmentionables!"

The group erupted again.

"Where were your shorts?" Grace asked, giggling.

"I had them!" Ruby cried. "He dropped 'em, and I grabbed 'em and swam back to the shore."

"So I was sent to bed after a thorough roastin' from my dad and no supper and no ice cream." Max shrugged, smiling widely, his dark eyes dancing in the firelight.

"How old were you?"

"Fourteen."

"Your first of many brushes with the law, huh?" Caleb commented. His tone wasn't condescending but there was an edge to it Grace couldn't place.

The deputy had been mostly quiet since their arrival and had only smiled briefly in Grace's direction after handing her a plate for her steak. He'd been close to the other of Buck's female friends for most of the day, while also helping Vince with the grill. Truthfully, Grace was relieved. He was nice enough, but his attention made her nervous. Not because she was scared of him. Far from it. He'd always been supernice and polite to her, offering to walk her home from the bar when she was on late shifts if Holly was out or Max wasn't around, which was rare. It was just that Max seemingly had a huge bee in his bonnet about the cop, and she didn't want to be responsible for a falling-out between the two men. Knowing herself, she'd be sure to say *something* wrong.

Max smirked at Caleb, but his stare across the licking flames of the bonfire was anything but pleasant. Grace shifted at his side, wanting to touch him, but not knowing how. "What's it to ya?"

Caleb shrugged and sipped his beer. "Just askin'."

Max opened his mouth to say something that Grace didn't doubt would be filled with expletives, but was interrupted by the sound of Journey blasting from the stereo Buck had brought. Buck leaped onto his seat and began his usual air guitar routine, along with Josh, who joined him and sang as loudly as he could about small-town girls and midnight trains. Before long everyone was singing, even Max, who laughed and encouraged Buck to jump like a true rock star from his seat.

They cheered and egged the boys on as they danced and goofed around. It was a shame that Grace had left her camera in her room. These were memories she wanted to document, to keep close to her heart, to look at whenever she was feeling bruised by life. She closed her eyes and allowed the sounds and smells of the moment to seep deeply into her, focusing on the gloriously loud laugh booming from Max's chest. Similar to hearing her favorite song, the sound of it sent rippling goose bumps all over her body like a wave around a baseball stadium.

Max moved close to Grace's ear when the song ended amid cheers and applause for Buck's performance and AC/DC's "Back in Black" began. "You okay?"

She smiled at Max's gentle nod as the legendary guitar riff echoed up the mountain. "Absolutely."

19

Grace was awoken by the sun streaming through a gap in the drapes and loud humming creeping from under the bathroom door. Grace rubbed her eyes and stretched. Her elbow bumped into the line of pillows that Max had been adamant about placing down the center of the bed. He stated their presence was to help make her feel safer, but something told Grace that Max needed those pillows between them, too—just for different reasons. Reasons that made her heart beat faster.

As she sat up and fastened her hair atop her head, the bathroom door opened and Max wandered out followed by a delicious-smelling cloud of steam. It was all deep spice and unlike any scent Grace had smelled before.

"Hey," he said with a smile, fastening the tie on his blue board shorts and pulling the hem of his white wifebeater back down, hiding the sliver of exposed sun-bronzed skin under his belly button. "You're awake."

He moved around the room quickly. The tattoo on his shoulder was more visible than Grace had seen since the day they'd touched in his room. Her heart squeezed at the memory. The tat was black, thick black that looked almost like flames, maybe feathers?

"Did you sleep well?" he asked, pulling on his watch and slipping on a pair of black flip-flops before running his hands through his damp hair. Grace kind of loved that he never seemed to use a brush, especially when his hair stuck up that way.

"Yeah," she replied, standing up and neatening the covers. "Did you?"

"Sure." He shrugged. "I sleep good anywhere there's a horizontal surface, ya know?"

Grace smiled, shuddering under the way his eyes traveled lazily down her cami top and sleep shorts. "Can I use the shower?" she asked, reaching for the towel folded on top of her bag.

"Yeah, of course. Buck, Josh, and I are gonna head down to the lake and set up the float and shit, maybe get the boat out. It'd be cool to spend the day on the water. It's hot. Come down and join us when you're ready. Uncle Vince is on breakfast duty."

She nodded, holding the towel close. "We're swimming today?"

Max flashed her a look that slid under her skin and made her warm. "We sure are. And you"—he took a large step toward her—"need to get that swimsuit on and show off that gorgeous body of yours." His top teeth pressed into his bottom lip. "It'd be a damned travesty if you didn't."

"Oh, well, I—" she flustered, her cheeks heating. "I— Yeah, I mean, okay, I might."

Max plucked his Ray-Ban shades from off the top of the dresser and slid them on. "That's my girl."

Without another word, he left the room, closing the door gently behind him. The three words he'd spoken wrapped around Grace like a warm hug and sent her heart into a very confusing frenzy.

• • • •

"Hey, Grace!" Ruby waved maniacally from where she stood at the water's edge. "Come over here, honey!"

Max was right: It was scorching hot. Grace's skin tingled under the sun's rays as she made her way to where the women of the house had set up their own little sun-worshipping oasis. Towels, loungers, beach umbrellas, and coolers were all in attendance, while the shouts and splashes Grace could hear alerted her to the fact that all the boys were in the lake doing . . . something.

"They're arguin' about floats and damn float fasteners," Ruby said with an eye roll. "We may never see them again." The red of Ruby's two-piece made her gray eyes pop, with not a muffin top in sight.

Grace glanced down at herself, suddenly conscious of the lush bodies around her. The swimsuit she was wearing was a yellow one-piece, a color that had always suited her. Yellow brought out the dark, warm tones of her skin, her momma had said. She'd bought her new swimsuit in haste two days before the trip to the cabin and hadn't tried it on until it was too late to take it back.

The legs were cut high, showing a couple of the scars on her hip, while the back was low, showing glimpses of the scars on her side. That's why she'd thrown on a thin white T-shirt she'd found crumpled on top of Max's bag. She hoped he didn't mind her borrowing his clothes, but the thought of walking around just in her suit dried her throat.

The T-shirt slipped down one shoulder and she'd tied it in a loose knot at her hip, leaving a small sliver of the lower half of her swimsuit showing. She'd never worn so little around other people, and outside to boot. Months ago, she'd never have dreamed of being so daring. She remembered wearing a bikini in her backyard one burning summer day. Rick had come home high and pissed and had beaten her with his shoe when he found her. He'd called her a whore because who knows who could have seen her flashing her slutty ass all over the place.

Their yard was private. No one had seen. But Rick's paranoia was a devastating thing.

"Maybe I should change?" she murmured suddenly, reaching for the shades on her head. Ruby's hand on hers was as surprising as it was a relief.

"No. Don't. You look incredible."

"You sure do," Carla added. "Girl, if I had legs like yours, I'd wear that outfit all the time."

Okay, so maybe this chick wasn't *too* bad, even if she did have a full face of makeup in one-hundred-degree heat. As long as she kept her eyes off Max, Grace would get along with her juuuuust fine. Her sudden possessiveness over Max was neither surprising nor worrying. It was in her nature. She'd always been that way with family, friends, boyfriends . . .

Grace looked out over the water at the sound of Vince's voice in the middle of the lake. She immediately spotted Max, shades still in place, shirtless and wet from the water, grinning at Buck as he tried to get the float to stay in place. Good God the man was dangerous. He truly was a vision. Unshaven, board shorts low, his lean runner's body kissed by the sun. Grace wanted to kiss him. She wanted to kiss him all over. She imagined he'd taste divine, if the smells he left in the shower were anything to go by.

"Beer?" Ruby asked, holding a bottle of Heineken up to Grace's nose.

Grace glanced at her watch. It was eleven thirty. "Sure. Why not? It's five o'clock somewhere, right?"

"That's what we like," Max's aunt Fern commented as she approached wearing a bikini top and sarong, carrying what looked like a tray full of homemade Popsicles and Jell-O shots. There was no way there wasn't any alcohol in those bad boys. Things were going to get messy, and fast.

"That float looks like a damned house," Grace observed, sipping her beer and placing her bag on one of the loungers. The float was huge and could hold at least ten people. It was like a floating deck, complete with steps into the water.

"It's great, right?" Aunt Fern replied. "Vince and I bought that a few years ago. It's the envy of the lake, you know?"

Ruby snorted and shook her head at the same time an almighty splash echoed around the water. Five men, arms flying in the front crawl, shot toward the shore. Ruby screamed and yelled for her husband while Carla, her blonde hair shining in the sun, called out Buck's name. Carla's friend—Anna? Ada?—smiled.

"Hey, Adele," Carla called over her shoulder to the brown-haired woman.

That's right. Adele.

"Looks like your man's in the lead."

"Shut up," Adele retorted, closing her large hazel eyes and lying back on her lounger, her flat stomach unblemished and toned in her blue two-piece. "It was one lousy kiss. It's not like I slept with the guy."

Grace frowned at Ruby in question, who mouthed, "Caleb."

Ah. Clearly, there'd been some shenanigans after she and Max had gone to bed. Interesting.

Max strode from the water, ribbing Buck about kicking his ass in the water again and pushing his black hair back from his forehead. His whole body shifted in a way that Grace had only ever seen on predator nature programs. Like a wildcat or something, he was all sinewy and sensual. Christ. She pressed her beer bottle to her cheek; the sun was already getting to her and her libido. What was it about the summer that had everyone's lustometer on high alert?

Max smirked as he approached. "You made it. Did you get some food?" He cocked an eyebrow at her clothing and lifted the hem of the T-shirt to her ribs. "This looks familiar."

"Yeah," Grace answered, quickly pushing it back down. She lowered her voice. "I hope you don't mind. I saw it on your bag and it covers up the parts that I don't want—you know, my skin where— I'll wash it and—"

Her ramblings were stopped by Max's fingers on her lips. He chuckled. "It's fine. Whatever you're comfortable in." He lifted his fingers and looked her over. "Remember, they're what you survived."

And just like that, Grace's breath vanished.

"Hey, Max, you wanna give me a hand over here, man?"

Max turned and headed toward where Josh was standing with a selection of chairs and water-friendly toys, making Grace gasp. The tattoo she'd seen on Max's shoulder was a tiny part of a piece of artwork that stretched right across from one shoulder to the other like angel's wings. Black feathers, so detailed they looked almost real, reached out across his skin, meeting at his spine and running all the way down to the small of his back, where the name Christopher curved in an arch, under which was a date and the words "ad infinitum."

Apart from the black, which Grace had seen previously, no other part of the tattoo extended to the front of his body. Like an inked secret few knew about, Max's tattoo was as beautiful as he was and posed even more questions.

Grace pressed her lips together and sat down, kicking off her flats and settling to watch the boys finish setting up. She knew the questions would have to wait. Today was about fun and sunshine in all their forms.

. . . .

"You gonna come into the water at all today?"

Max stood at the foot of Grace's lounger with a bottle of Pepsi in his hand, admiring her long legs and despairing over the fact that, in three hours, she'd still not taken his fucking shirt off or joined them on the float. On top of that, the fact that she'd chosen to wear a piece of his clothing had caused his stomach to twist and his groin to twitch. Yeah, that was hot. The other guys had commented on how hot it was, too. Except Deputy AssFlap, who'd rolled his eyes in blatant jealousy. Well, he could just suck a dick. Or let that brunette do it and get it all out of his system.

Max flicked the cold moisture from his soda bottle onto Grace's foot, making her jump and look up from her cell phone.

She laughed. "Hey!" She wiped her foot. "I'm okay here," she said softly. "I'm happy playing Angry Birds. Honestly. Go and have fun. I love the sun. I'm good." She shrugged and scrunched up her nose.

Yeah, she'd started to catch the sun, too. Her dark skin had already begun to change color. Highlights at her hairline shone bright caramel and gold. She also looked a little buzzed, which was cute as hell. Max knew that his aunt Fern and Ruby had made sure she'd always had a fresh drink at her side.

"But everyone's out on the float now," he pointed out. "You're all on your own."

"Max, I'm okay. I promise."

He huffed. "Well, will you at least come here while I show you something?" he asked, kicking a foot at one of the lounger legs.

She cocked a suspicious eyebrow. "Something?"

He smirked. "Not *that* something." He waggled his eyebrows. "Not now, at least."

She laughed and sat forward. "Okay. What do you want to show me?"

"Come here."

Placing her cell on the lounger, she moved closer, standing carefully but unable to completely stop the slight sway in her gait. She giggled. "Those Jell-O shots are naughty."

"I hear ya," Max replied with a chuckle. "Hey," he said frowning. "What's that?" He pointed to her feet.

As she looked down, Max made his move. As though she weighed nothing, he grabbed her around the tops of her thighs and hiked her over his shoulder in a firefighter's lift, grinning as cheers of encouragement erupted from the bastards on the float who'd dared him to do it. He hurried down toward the water, ignoring Grace's squeals of protest, the tone of her voice thick with humor, and until he heard her panic, he wasn't letting go.

"Max! I swear to God! Let me down." She smacked his ass. Hard.

"Oh, you can do that again," he retorted, wading into the water. She shrieked when it touched her toes. It would no doubt feel fucking bitter against her hot skin. "I've got you," he hummed. "Don't you worry."

"Oh my heavens, it's freezing, Max! Stop!"

Max chuckled. Even with liquor in her, she was still careful about cursing.

"Stop?" he asked, and halted his steps immediately, the water lapping at his waist.

"Thank you," she gasped. "Now let me down."

He grinned toward the float. "Okay. I'll let you down. Here's a good spot."

With ease and a piercing scream from Grace as he did, Max lifted her and threw her into the water. The whole of her submerged. He bowed and waved at the float, where everyone was on his or her feet, laughing, whistling, and applauding.

"You bastard!" Grace spluttered as she broke the surface and stood up, hair dripping, white T-shirt clinging deliciously to her body. She flailed her hands, as if the movement would help in her effort to get dry.

Max moved toward her, grinning. "Oh, come on now. Don't be mad." He reached out. "My clothes never looked so fucking good."

She smirked. "Is that right?"

His eyes danced down her body, paying particularly close attention to her hard nipples. "Shit yeah," he breathed, thankful that the water was cold enough to keep his cock at bay.

"Well," she purred. "Come closer and tell me more."

Max should have listened to his gut. He should have listened to the sensible part of his brain and not the part of his brain that resided in his shorts, because as soon as he moved closer she was on him, dunking him headfirst into the lake, over and over again, winding her lithe body around his until he was begging for mercy. She was like a slippery eel. Max simply couldn't get a hold on her, but Jesus, having her body so close, so near nakedness was fucking stupendous. Her thighs gripped him tightly while his cheek pressed into her tit.

Awesome.

She finally let go, pushing away with a laugh that was beautiful. "I have a brother, Maxie," she taunted while swimming backward. "Don't forget. I learned from the best. I dunk boys like you for breakfast."

And with that she took off toward the float, where Josh and Buck helped her climb aboard, leaving Max tongue-tied and bursting with pride.

20

It was late afternoon when everyone left the float for the shade of the house. With the sun still hot as hell and drinks being thrown back like nobody's business, a siesta was in serious order. With an arm behind his head and a foot on the ground to keep the hammock, tied between two trees, swinging gently, Max watched Grace approach with a soft, tipsy smile across her sun-kissed face. She was still wearing his godforsaken T-shirt, but that was okay. She'd been nothing but an absolute pleasure to be around all day, opening up to him and everyone else, shaking off her natural timidity and quiet.

He smiled when she stopped at his side. "Hi."

"Hi," she answered. "You okay?"

He nodded. "You?"

She lifted her half-empty bottle of water. "Trying to dilute. I may be a little buzzed."

"I think you just might be." He patted the hammock. "Wanna join me?"

She frowned. "There's room?"

Max shifted, leaving a small space for her. "There is now."

Grace placed her water on the ground and, with zero elegance, sat down heavily on the hammock's edge, pushing it sideways sharply and causing her to fall back onto Max.

"Oh shit!" he exclaimed.

A loud, dirty laugh burst from her as Max, with flailing arms and legs, attempted to steady the damn thing and keep them both on top of it. He managed, just, despite Grace not helping one bit.

With them both lying back, Grace still wheezing with laughter, Max shook his head.

"You're nuts," he commented with a wry smile.

"I feel nuts," she replied, placing a hand on her chest in an effort to calm herself. "I feel great." She looked over at him, their noses mere inches apart. "I love it here. I've had such a good time."

"I'm glad." Max's gaze did a slow circuit of her face. "You've caught the sun."

"You, too." She pressed her index finger to his nose. "You have freckles."

"I do not!"

Grace giggled again. "Don't worry, they're adorable."

Max rubbed his hands down his face in an attempt to rid himself of said adorableness. "Whatever."

She grinned and looked back at the sky, her hand grazing his. "It's been nice seeing you so happy."

He looked at her, surprised.

She closed her eyes. "Your smile is far too nice not to show off."

Without thought, Max pushed his arm under her head and pulled her close. The scent of sun-heated skin, sun screen, and wine filled his senses. "You're flirty when you drink, huh?"

Seemingly unfazed by his holding her, she nodded. "Apparently." She opened one eye. "Does that bother you?"

Max shook his head. "It's adorable."

She laughed and moved her hand so that it rested on his bare stomach. His muscles immediately clenched. He cleared his throat. "You kept my T-shirt on."

Grace hummed in reply. "You have a tattoo."

He sighed. "I do."

Grace's eyes opened slowly, their prior haziness fading to something more sensitive. "Wanna talk about it?"

Did he want to talk about it? Not really. But Max knew there would come a time when he would have to open up, to tell people about his past and what he'd been through. Who better to start with than Grace, with her innocent questions and open face. Besides, she'd shared such a dark and painful part of herself when she told him about Rick.

"Christopher was my son," he said quietly, the words scratching his throat like fractured pieces of his heart slipping up from his chest.

Grace became very still. The only movement the gentle sway of the hammock. "Was."

Max turned his head, looking straight at her. "He died."

A small breath escaped Grace's lips. She pulled her hand away from his stomach but he clasped her wrist quickly.

"Don't," he urged. He placed it back, needing the contact while he told his story, the story of Christopher, the story of Lizzie, the story of why he'd taken the path he had and why he was the way he was.

Grace stayed silent throughout, her fingers moving ever so slightly against his skin when he described losing Christopher and then Lizzie. The drugs, the drinking, the women, all of it spewed from him as they lay on his father's hammock under the shade of the trees.

It was minutes after he'd finished before Grace spoke. "I'm so very sorry, Max."

He shrugged. "Don't be."

"How could she just leave you like that?" She lifted onto her elbow, looking down at him, and moved her hand to his heart, pressing carefully. "This has been hurt so much."

"S'why it doesn't work anymore." He licked his lips and his eyelids fluttered closed when her fingers whispered across his nipple.

"Sure it does," she retorted with a gentle shake of her head. "You just don't realize it." Her hand traveled down the center of his chest, pausing briefly at his belly button. "You're very special, Max."

He gripped her waist gently, hoping to God that she'd move her hand farther down. Despite the gravity of the conversation they'd just had, his need for her touch was overwhelming.

"Gracie." Her stare remained glued to the waistband of his shorts and the undeniable shape of his cock, as it grew hard under her attention. "Touch me."

Gradually her hand shifted, over the material of his shorts, over his erection, drawing a hiss from his lips. Her touch was tentative, careful, causing Max to lift his hips to chase a firmer grip, a rougher stroke.

"That's it," he encouraged, rubbing his palm down her back. "That's it."

His words seemed to light her confidence, as she pressed against him harder, gripping him. Although the feel of her was amazing, Max's body moved with ripples of frustration, wanting her to push his clothes away and jerk him hard. But he didn't push. Instead, he pulled down the front of the T-shirt she wore as well as the edge of her swimsuit and sucked eagerly on her nipple, earning a deep moan from her throat. Her nipples were as dark as chocolate and, just as they had before, pebbled perfectly against his tongue. As he had hoped, Grace's hand gripped him harder, rubbing stronger until his hips and hers were writhing, seeking out more friction, to make the hammock sway.

"Let me touch you," Max gasped into her neck, the salt on her sweet skin driving him beyond distraction. "Fuck, let me put my fingers in you."

"God." Her head fell back at his words, leaving him to lick and suck up to her ear and down to her collarbone.

Taking her reaction as permission, Max moved his hand to her thigh, noting how soft she felt, pulling it toward him, and opening her up. "I'll be gentle," he promised around a grunt as she continued working him, drawing an orgasm from deep in the depths of his stomach. His fingers skimmed the damp material between her legs, making her body jump.

"I've got you. I'm gonna make it so fucking good, so—"

"Max?" Josh's shout came from by the water, from beyond the trees where no one could see them, but it brought them both to a screeching halt all the same. "You out here?"

Max cursed and pulled his hands from between Grace's legs, while she flustered and moved so quickly away from him that once again the hammock tilted dangerously, leaving them both flapping to keep on it.

Josh emerged just as they had the damn thing under control. "Oh," he said, embarrassment tinging his cheeks. "Sorry, dude, I didn't realize—"

"It's okay," Max said with a hand up, even though it was the biggest damn lie he'd told. His groin pulsed with the remnants of his hard-on, which he prayed Josh didn't notice, while his heart thumped like a hammer in his chest. "What's up?"

Josh threw his thumb over his shoulder. "So we're all gonna go into town, have a few more drinks, maybe hit a club. Everyone's getting ready now. We're leaving in about thirty. You in?"

Almost.

Max glanced at Grace, taking in her flushed cheeks and aroused eyes. "You up for it?"

"Sure," she said a little too quickly, in a voice that was husky and filled with desire. "Sounds good."

"We'll be there," Max said with a salute toward Josh, who turned quickly and jogged back the way he came.

Max rubbed a hand across his forehead. "Well, that'll give Ruby something to talk about for the next million years."

Grace groaned and dropped her head to his shoulder. "She'll never let me live this down."

Max patted her hair before gently moving away. She was altogether too fucking tempting with her heat, scent, and willingness, and they'd never be ready in time if they started again. He stood carefully from the hammock and stretched his arms above his head.

When he turned back, Grace's eyes were all over him and all about the sex.

"Jesus," he muttered into his palm with a smile. "Stop it, or we'll never leave."

"What?" she asked with an innocent blink.

"You know what." He laughed, offering her his hand, which she took without pause. "Come on, let's get ready. I need a cold shower."

. . . .

The shower Max took was frigid. Still, he seriously deliberated about whacking one out. Knowing Grace was in the next room all sweet and oblivious to her sexiness, however, made him equal parts exhilarated and uneasy about the prospect. After much debate, he decided against it and tried his best to think unsexy thoughts— rehab, Tate, therapy—which worked wonderfully until, after dressing, he walked back into the room to find Grace leaning over her suitcase in nothing but her underwear.

Sweet Jesus.

Her ass looked freaking spectacular, cupped by red lace that accentuated the caramel tone of her skin. He slumped against the doorjamb, stunned by the lascivious images that were suddenly flashing through his brain.

Apparently, he made a noise of appreciation, because Grace abruptly spun around with a sound of surprise, using her arms and hands to try to hide the red lace bra and panty set she wore. But that shit was futile. Max had seen all he needed to bring his body roaring back to ready, set, let's fuck.

He tried to be a gentleman, truly he did, but his eyes betrayed him on every level, skating across her thighs, her waist, before seeking out that luscious mystery between her legs. He cleared his throat, mumbled an apology, and wandered across the bedroom, finding a spot that was as far away from her as possible. When he turned back, she was clutching a towel to her body, looking as aroused as he was feeling.

After a moment of tense silence, a laugh of incredulity burst from him. "Shit, woman, you're killing me."

"I'm sorry, I was in a world of my own and I thought you'd be longer in there and—" Grace paused for a moment before creasing into infectious giggles. "Oh my God, your face."

Max couldn't help but laugh with her and it felt so damned good. "Mine? What about yours?"

He shook his head. He felt totally unbalanced around her, he lacked control, all sense eluded him, yet, instead of it causing any anxiety, he found himself embracing it. Her spontaneity and apparent amusement at his enduring desire for her were fresh and new, leaving a sensation of something that felt suspiciously like happiness creeping through the dark crevasses of his soul.

She snorted and breathed deeply, trying to regain some sort of calm while wafting her hands by her face. "I've just done my mascara, dammit!"

"Okay, well, I'll go down to hang with the guys while you finish"—he motioned toward her—"you know, dressing."

Grace coughed a laugh. "Okay."

Running his hands through his hair in a fruitless attempt to delete the images invading his mind, Max found his uncle and Josh sitting by the bar in the sitting room. Both men whispered heatedly, clearly up to shit, but sat up straight, shutting up quickly when they saw Max approach. Bastards. Uncle Vince cocked a suspicious eyebrow and opened his mouth to speak.

Max held up a hand. "Don't think because you're old I won't beat you," he said simply, to which both men boomed with laughter. Max took a seat next to them, smiling.

"Well, at least a hammock is creative," Uncle Vince muttered around the lip of his beer bottle. "Even your aunt and I haven't tried that."

Both Josh and Max groaned in distaste before the latter dropped his head to his forearm. His uncle slapped his back. "Oh, come on, Maxie, lighten up! When was the last time I got to rib you about getting fresh with a girl, huh? Let me have my fun!" He turned his eyes back to Josh. "I remember when his father and I caught him with this girl at the back of his shop."

A disbelieving laugh exploded out of Max. "Really? We're still on that?"

"Absofreakinlutely we are, boy." His uncle pressed a finger to the bar top. "Until I can't speak no more, we'll be on this!"

Josh chuckled. "What happened?"

Uncle Vince looked far too excited for Max's taste. "Well, Max's daddy and I were—"

"Seriously?" Max complained through a smile.

"—working on this hot as hell Corvette, when Connor noticed that Max had disappeared." He shrugged. "Wouldn't have bothered Connor usually, he let Max have a lot of freedom, but Max should have been helping out at the shop as part of his punishment for something else he'd done. Little shit was always in some sort of trouble." His words were truth, but he smiled fondly at Max.

Josh grinned. "Where was he?"

"He being me?" Max asked, lifting a hand. "I *am* sitting here."

Without turning, Uncle Vince waved him off. "Had this little blonde thing pressed up against the hood of his daddy's Mustang and was struggling to unfasten her damn bra!"

"It was a front fastener!" Max argued with arms wide at his sides. "How the hell was I supposed to know?"

Uncle Vince snorted. "Connor and I must have stood there for a good minute listening to him curse the godforsaken thing before the girl spotted us." He and Josh laughed harder. "She upped and darted, flushing crimson and calling Max names even I'd never heard of."

"How old were you that you hadn't been introduced to front fastener bras?" Josh asked through his chuckles.

"Twenty-five," his uncle joked before Max could reply with the actual answer of sixteen.

Max found himself laughing at the memory while he poured himself a Dr Pepper. His father had been more concerned that there was an ass print on the hood of his prize Mustang than about his son trying to get laid with some girl. That same girl, Sarah Miller, had never even looked at him again after that. Not that Max had blamed her. In fact, if he remembered correctly, he was pretty sure Carter fucked her at a party not long afterward.

"Oh, to be young again," Uncle Vince mused. He nudged Max's shoulder and winked.

"Leave the boy alone, Vincent."

Max sighed in relief at the sound of Aunt Fern's voice. "They're bullying me *again,* Aunt Fern," he grumbled. "Tell them."

"Bullying." Uncle Vince mocked with a snort. He pointed at Max with his beer bottle. "Don't use my hammock for your nefarious plans and I won't!"

"Nefarious?" Max laughed. "Aunt Fern, I think Uncle Vince has been watching late-night TV again."

His aunt pointed a stern finger at her husband and son-in-law. "You two be nice," she scolded. "Leave Max alone."

"Yeah," Max agreed with a sharp dip of his chin, placing one hand on his aunt's shoulder in unity while using the other to lift his drink to his mouth. "Leave me alone."

Aunt Fern smiled wide. "He's in love, it's sweet."

The Dr Pepper Max was drinking projected from his mouth in a disbelieving spray across the bar, narrowly missing the laughing people sitting next to it.

"What?" he spluttered, wiping his mouth with the back of his hand. "Aunt Fern! Grace and I, we're not— It's not what you think, we're . . ."

Her hand patting his cheek stopped his ramblings. "So cute."

Josh's laughter raised in volume. "Dude, this is awesome."

Max shot him a look that said that this was unequivocally *not* awesome.

"What's all the racket?" Ruby came bounding into the room, wineglass in hand, followed by Buck, his girlfriends, and Deputy AssCrack.

"Your father and husband are assholes," Max murmured, still wiping his face.

Ruby sniggered. "That's not news."

"What's not news?"

Max looked up when he heard Grace's soft voice from the doorway and for one split second he forgot that he wanted to throttle Josh for gossiping and his uncle for telling embarrassing stories. She stood there, fidgeting yet lovely. Her hair was down, black and thick with a couple of short baby curls crafted perfectly to her temples. The red and white floral dress she wore skimmed her thighs and dipped between her boobs, hugging her figure in ways that were tastefully sexy. She approached him slowly, the glint in her eye suggesting that, just like him, their heavy petting session was still the only thing she could think about.

A shiver of pride ran through him. Yeah, he thought to himself, *he* was the man who she was fooling around with. He was the man who she trusted to make her come and feel good. He was the man she wanted to touch her and teach her how to be intimate again.

Shit, if he'd had feathers he'd have preened like a motherfucker.

"You look great," he said when she reached him.

She brushed a hand down the dress and gave a modest shrug. "Thanks." She turned to him, her face pinching. "Hey, I wanted to ask you something." She glanced around and spoke when she seemed satisfied that no one but Max was listening. "Are you going to be okay going out tonight?"

Max's frown creased. "Sure." He lifted his shoulders. "Why wouldn't I be?"

She cleared her throat. "It's just, I was thinking. I know you hang out at Whiskey's a lot, but that's different. I mean, will you be all right going to a club?" Her big green eyes were worried. "You know, there'll be more . . . temptation. Are you okay with that? I'd be happy to stay here with you if not. We could watch a movie or something."

No one except Tate and Elliot had really asked Max about his addiction and what he could and couldn't manage in terms of the lures around him. Max knew it wasn't because his family and friends didn't care; they simply trusted him enough and believed in him enough to leave him to his own devices. His vice had never been alcohol as much as cocaine, but he knew how quickly one addiction could be filled with another. Plus he couldn't drink while on his meds. His steps helped, of course, but Max understood how cautious people were, of asking too much or coddling him, which he hated. But, apparently, Grace being cautious was an altogether different thing and caused a tug in Max's chest that was warm and comforting.

He smiled gently. "Grace, I'll be fine. The clubs around here aren't like the ones I went to in New York. I doubt there'll be too much to worry about. Besides, I'm the designated driver."

She nodded, looking down at the floor, appearing embarrassed. "Oh. Okay. I just thought I'd ask. I didn't want you to be uncomfortable."

Max moved closer, subtly running the tip of his index finger along her forearm. "Thank you," he murmured. "For caring enough to ask."

She lifted her face to his. "You're welcome."

·   ·   ·

The club was absolutely nothing like the dives Max used to frequent in the city. This place played pop music and had disco balls hanging from the ceiling, for shit's sake.

Max side-eyed Josh in annoyance. "What the fuck?"

Josh shrugged drunkenly in response just as Ruby squealed when some heinous boy-band music started blaring from the DJ stand. She grabbed Josh's arm and dragged the poor bastard across the club so she could dance with him. Max glanced around, fighting down the urge to bolt.

The walls were adorned with mirrors and pictures of musicians from every era from the sixties to the present day, including Britney Spears and the other blonde chick who wore chaps with her ass on show, next to a picture of a leather-clad Elvis. Poor dude was probably turning in his grave. It was hell on earth. Max knew that if Carter heard about his being in such a place, he'd have ended their friendship immediately. And Max wouldn't have blamed him. Even Buck looked forlorn dressed in his Van Halen T-shirt and Vans. While the girls, including his aunt, jumped and flailed to the beat around Josh, Max placed himself at the bar next to his uncle and the deputy and watched.

The place was bustling, filled with Independence Day revelers, some dressed in costumes ranging from Mickey Mouse to Darth Vader, making the atmosphere light. People smiled, hugged, and generally looked like they were having an awesome time, which helped Max stop thinking about the fact that he was nursing a Pepsi and not a shot of something stronger. Not that he'd thought about it all that much. In truth, all night his mind had been on one particular woman on the dance floor, looking spectacular as she lifted her arms and sang ABBA at the top of her lungs. He smiled. Max was certainly seeing another side to Grace. With each drink she consumed, she became chattier, more tactile, and a lot flirtier. She was definitely testing Max's resolve, but he found himself enjoying her attentions.

"She's a pretty girl."

Max looked from the dancing to his uncle and back again. "Don't start."

His uncle chuckled and moved closer. "Who's starting?"

Max snorted. "It's not like that between us." He saw his uncle in his periphery, nodding as he drank from his beer glass. "We're friends."

"She doesn't look at you like you're just her friend, Max."

Max turned to look at the man at his side, his smile fading at the cautious tone in his uncle's voice. He wasn't exactly sure what Uncle Vince's words made him feel, but there was definitely a pinch of something that felt suspiciously like panic at the base of his neck.

"Look," Uncle Vince continued, turning to face the bar instead of the dance floor, shoulder to shoulder with Max. "I don't wanna know what's going on between you two. It's not my business. You look happy together, friends or more. I just want to make sure that she treats you right. That shit there *is* my business."

Max blinked. "Treats *me* right?" He barked a laugh. "Shouldn't that be the other way around?"

His uncle didn't answer with anything other than a pointed look. "You're fragile, Max. You hide it well, but I can see it because I've known you since your daddy put you in my arms when you were two days old." Max shuffled uncomfortably while his uncle glanced back toward the dance floor. "She cares for you, but so did Lizzie." Max swallowed hard, his throat tight. "All's I'm saying is be careful, son. Don't lose yourself in something you're not ready for. Wouldn't be fair on either of you."

Max nodded. "It's all good," he assured his uncle. "Honestly. We both know where we stand. I'll be careful."

Uncle Vince placed a large hand on Max's shoulder and squeezed. "That's all I wanted to hear."

A collection of excited squeals had the two men's heads snapping back to the dance floor as the familiar opening bars of "Ain't No Mountain High Enough" filled the club. Well, Max thought, as the girls started jumping around even more, at least this song was an improvement on the shit that had been played since they arrived. In fact, he had this particular song on vinyl. It had been his mom's. His dad had told him once that, while she was pregnant with him, Max's mom would listen to it at least once a day, singing and stroking her baby bump. He was sure that somewhere in his apartment back in New York, he had a photograph that his dad had given him of her doing it.

The small smile that pulled at his lips at the memory grew wider when he saw Grace dancing, well, jumping toward him. She looked ridiculously endearing, all wide eyes and hair flying about. And the dress? Yeah, the dress was still fucking tremendous. Max had noticed the lingering stares it coaxed from the other guys in the bar but tried his best to ignore the shameless flash of possessiveness that streaked through him. His stink-eye was enough to keep those dipshits at bay.

"Come and dance!" she shouted above the music when she reached him, just as Marvin Gaye sang about remembering the day. Before Max could answer, Grace grabbed his hand and started swinging it from side to side, miming the words and bopping like a damn rabbit from foot to foot.

Unable to resist her happy face and happier dancing, Max lifted his arm so she could twirl beneath it. She beamed. "My love is alive way down in my heart!" she sang loudly while wiggling her ass.

It took a moment for Max to realize that he was dancing, too, just a little, rocking from one foot to the other. Once again Grace's infectious spirit had yanked him away from any worries that his uncle may have had, any temptations and melancholy memories. Throwing caution to the wind and losing himself in the chorus of his mother's favorite song, he wrapped an arm around Grace's waist, gripped her free hand in the other, and began dancing—silly dancing—with her. He tipped her backward, swayed her from side to side, and twirled her some more. Her loud laugh filled the room over the music as he did and, whether he realized it or not, slowly crept into the deep, cold recesses of Max's heart.

. . .

At a little after one in the morning, with pizzas, burgers, and fries bought and devoured in the car on the way back to the house, Max held on to a very tipsy Grace as she stumbled up the stairs to their bedroom. She giggled and hummed to herself as she leaned on his arm, while repeating how much of an amazing, fantastic, truly *amazing* night she'd had. Max couldn't help but laugh at her. Truth was she was stinking cute when she was drunk.

"And the fireworks?" she slurred. "Oh my gosh, they're so pretty. So pretty. Did you see them?"

"I saw them."

"They were pretty, right? And all boom and pfffftttttt!" She flailed her arms to show Max just how pretty the fireworks were and tilted sideways.

Max held her tightly while he pushed open the door, glad that she barely weighed anything when she slumped her entire body against him. "Pretty like you," she mumbled into his bicep as they moved into the room.

Max snorted. "You're not gonna puke, are you?" he asked as she staggered toward the bed and dropped onto it face-first like a starfish, hair surrounding her like a black halo. She held wobbly thumbs up in answer.

Max checked out the way her dress gathered high on the backs of her thighs and rubbed a hand down his face. "I'm gonna wash up, okay?"

The comforter muffled her answer. "Mkay."

In the bathroom, standing with his hands on the sink, Max thought back to what his uncle had said in the club. He shouldn't have been surprised by his uncle's concerns. Max himself had gone through the whole should he, shouldn't he circle in his head about whether doing whatever the hell it was that he was doing with Grace was a sound idea.

And he was still convinced it was.

They were two—granted, fucked-up—consenting adults who found each other attractive. They were fuck buddies and nothing more. Yet both Tate and his uncle had pointed out that Grace may have *wanted* more, liked Max more than she should.

Max stared at himself in the mirror. "Shit."

If he was truly honest with himself, Max liked Grace. He liked her a lot, but the scarred, battered, and bruised muscle that beat in his chest just wasn't up to the task of loving anyone ever again.

The last thing he wanted to do was hurt her. She deserved more than that. It wasn't that Max thought Grace loved him. No. Despite Tate's and his uncle's words, Max knew better. She may have looked at him with affection, but that was merely because she showed her feelings without any filter. She was like an open book and, ironically enough, that was one thing Max really liked about her. There was no bullshit. She said it how it was.

And then there was the fact that he wanted her. Shit, of course he wanted her. He couldn't wait to be inside her and see if she'd go off like the firecracker he hoped for.

He'd been clear on his terms when they agreed to help each other, clear on what he was open and closed to, and Grace had accepted that. And not just accepted it, she'd been of the same damn opinion. He just had to trust that she could keep behind the lines they'd marked in the ground between themselves when they shook hands. Max really wasn't sure what he'd do if she didn't. Maybe they needed to talk about it.

Resolute, he pushed from the sink and opened the door back into the bedroom, losing all ability to think or fucking speak when he saw Grace lying on the bed, faceup, head on the pillows, in nothing but that damned red underwear. And fuck him sideways if it wasn't the hottest thing. He noticed her dress in a puddle by his feet along with her shoes.

She smiled, buzzed, her right hand meandering across her stomach. "Hey."

Max cleared his throat, his gaze devouring her from the tips of her toes to her tits. "Hey."

"You about done thinking so hard in there all by yourself?"

He pressed his lips together, fighting a smile. Oh, yeah. She was even feistier when she drank. He crossed his arms over his chest, because fuck, what else was there to do but look? "Maybe."

"Good." She nodded toward his crotch, where he knew he was sporting a righteous hard-on. "You gonna come over here with that?"

"Behave. I'm not fuckin' you while you're drunk."

"I know. Besides, I wasn't thinking about that," she murmured, her eyes closing while her fingertips whispered across her chest. *Sweet Jesus.*

"What *were* you thinking about?" Max took two steps toward the bed, pulling his T-shirt over his head and launching it across the room.

Grace hummed when she saw his chest and pressed her teeth into her bottom lip. "You're so beautiful."

"I guess beautiful is an improvement on pretty. How much have you drunk, exactly?"

She giggled. "Enough." Yeah, Max knew that. He'd been keeping a watch on every drink that she'd bought or had bought for her all night, making sure she was okay. She licked her lips. "Enough to know I want your hands on me."

Max kneeled on the bed by her feet. "Yeah?"

"Yeah. I want my hands on you, too."

Max reached out and trailed his palm up her shin. It was as smooth and as soft as he'd imagined. Her breath left her in a ragged whisper.

"Where would you want to touch me?" he asked. Her gaze drifted from his face to his jeans and as God was his fucking witness, Max's cock jumped. "I told you," he grunted, placing a hand on the outside of both of her feet. "Touch me wherever and whenever you want." He unfastened the button on his Levi's and slid the zipper down, showing a glimpse of gray underwear. He leaned forward and placed a kiss on the inside of Grace's knee. She whimpered. He did it again and she moaned at the same time her legs dropped open.

Fuck, he just wanted to bury his face in her, lose himself for days in her wet and heat. Instead he kissed her inner thigh, noting the way her breathing hitched. She never flinched. He did it again and she arched her back. "Oh, God."

Max hummed into her skin, smelling and tasting that damn cocoa butter that he liked so much. His tongue traveled the inside of her thigh.

"Oh, God," she repeated, her hands shifting on the bed.

"You're okay," Max whispered, rubbing a gentle hand against her stomach.

"No, I—"

"I've got you, it's okay."

"No, Max."

He nuzzled the crease where her thigh met her hip. "Tell me what you want me to do."

"Move. I need you to move."

"Move?"

"I'm going to be sick."

Max sat up as though his ass were on fire, narrowly dodging Grace's swinging arms and legs as she dropped clumsily off the side of the bed and veered into the bathroom, smacking into the door-jamb before making it through and emitting the most fuck-awful gagging noise Max had ever heard.

After a beat of disbelief, he cupped a hand to his forehead. Talk about a libido killer. He looked down at himself and his now half-flaccid cock and grunted. "Jesus," he muttered while clambering off the bed and zipping himself back up. He peeked around the door of the bathroom and saw Grace kneeling on the floor, head in the throat of the toilet. "You okay?"

She groaned. "No." She sniffed and heaved some more.

Approaching cautiously, Max gathered her hair that splayed down her back as well as the parts that had fallen forward in her haste to get to the john and sat on the edge of the bathtub, holding it clear of any rogue chunks.

"Crap, I'm sorry," she garbled before she hurled again.

Max chuckled at the sight of her in her sexy underwear, up-chucking the night's festivities. "Don't worry about it." Of course, it wasn't how he'd imagined tonight to go, but that didn't matter.

Keeping her hair in one hand, he rubbed her back softly with the other.

21

Rhinos.

Rhinos, elephants, and any other large, stampeding-type mammals had obviously invaded Grace's bedroom last night and jumped all over her head. How else could she explain the horrific pain that wrapped her entire skull and the grotesque throbbing going on behind her eyelids? Seriously. Her eyes had a damned pulse.

She cracked one open, immediately hating the glorious sunshine that pierced her pupils. Christ Almighty, it had been a very long time since she'd drunk so much. Truth be told it had been a very long time since she'd been relaxed enough to enjoy herself to such a degree. And enjoy herself she had. She moved sluggishly, lifting her head gingerly from the pillow, realizing quickly that she was wearing only her underwear and that she was alone in the bed. And no wonder, the smell of stale alcohol and vomit lingered around the room.

Oh, Lord, the fool she had made of herself last night! Flashes of Max's magnificent chest and the feel of his luscious mouth against her raced through her mind, sending her into another merry-go-round of dizziness. She'd been so sure with all those cocktails still swilling around inside her that seducing Max was, at the time, the most epic of ideas. Puking mid-foreplay, however, had not been part of her audacious plan.

"Nicely played, Grace," she muttered to herself, lifting the covers and dropping her legs off the side of the bed. Dammit, he'd even held her hair back while she puked. Her face heated with embarrassment. Exhaling despondently, she noticed a glass of water on the side table, and next to it two pills that looked suspiciously like Tylenol. Grace's chest fluttered. Max was always considerate, but it never failed to make her all warm and fuzzy inside.

She knocked them back before staggering to the bathroom and the shower, hoping to God that the warm water would help wash away the shame of the previous night.

•   •   •

By the time Grace had washed and dressed herself in shorts and a vest top, everyone was either by the lake sunning themselves, swimming, or, like Ruby and Josh, playing tennis. Ruby didn't even look like she'd seen an alcoholic drink, let alone matched Grace cocktail for cocktail all night. Damn her. Max was nowhere in sight. She exhaled a breath of relief, not quite ready to face him.

Aunt Fern, Carla, and Adele looked over from their loungers as she approached, smiling gamely.

"You're up!" Adele said with a grin.

"Hey! Hey! Dancing girl's here!" Buck called from the water, where he stood with Caleb, who smiled widely at her. Grace waved in humiliation. "Let's start this party!" Buck added.

Carla glanced at her watch. It was past noon. "I knew all that dancing would tire you out."

"Yeah," Grace answered, vaguely remembering that she and Carla had become super best friends over the course of the night, conveying each other's awesomeness as more and more drinks were consumed. Apparently, she wasn't quite the bitch Grace had originally considered her to be. "I think the alcohol helped, too."

All three women laughed before Adele offered a lounger, which Grace took gratefully.

"We've all eaten. Can I fix you something, honey?" Aunt Fern asked.

Grace's stomach rolled at the mere thought. "No. Thank you." She held up her bottle of water. "I'm good."

Lying down helped. Grace sat back and closed her eyes behind her shades, enjoying the warmth and the sounds of splashing water and laughter. Despite her heinous hangover, she allowed the calm and contentment that encircled her to soak in. It was as close to peace as Grace had felt in a long time, surrounded by good people—friends—who accepted her without question.

A low, appreciative whistle conjured Grace's eyes open. "Goddamn, girl, I'd give my high teeth for a piece of that ass." Adele looked over at her. "Please, tell me you're hitting the shit out of that."

Grace followed Adele's admiring gaze to see Max and his uncle running up the shore toward them. Max was shirtless and had clearly worked up a sweat. It glistened and enhanced the grooves of his chest and stomach. His whole body tensed and flexed as he moved, muscles working hard, his cheeks blowing in and out, as he concentrated on each stride. He sure was a vision.

A deep warmth settled in Grace's stomach and between her legs. Dammit, who was she kidding? Adele was right; she should be hitting the shit out of that. She managed to school her features just as he slowed to a walk and approached her, sly smile in place, looking far too delicious with his chest heaving and black hair wet and clinging to his forehead. He ran a hand through it, making it stand in all different directions, and grabbed a bottle of water from the cooler.

"Well, good afternoon, Starshine," he said before he gulped at his drink. He swallowed and held the bottle to his cheek. "How's the head?"

She grimaced. "Fuzzy."

He chuckled and raised his eyebrows. "I'm sure it is. A gallon of cocktails will do that." He glanced over at Carla pointedly before fixing Grace with an intense stare. "What exactly do you remember from last night?"

She cleared her throat and pulled at the bottom of her top. "Bits and bobs . . . puking, dancing, being an idiot." She was hopelessly aware of there being three sets of curious eyes and ears watching and listening to their conversation. She sat up as if to lift herself from the lounger and removed her shades. "Can we talk?"

Max's face lost some of its playfulness. "Sure. I need a shower anyway." He looked over at his aunt. "Won't be long." He turned and made his way back to the house, Grace following close on his heels. They were halfway up the stairs to their room when he spoke again. "You all right apart from the hangover?"

She nodded. "Yeah, I just wanted to apologize."

Max stopped short by their bedroom door. "What for?"

Grace moved past him, entering the room with a loud sigh. She felt him follow and heard the door shut. "I'm sorry I did what I did." She reached the bed and turned to him, fisting her hands together, trying to find the right words. "It was silly and completely inappropriate."

Max stared at her for a beat and lifted his shoulders. "No problem."

"And I'm sorry for getting so drunk. It wasn't fair to you to have to deal with me being a drunken mess, especially with what you're *already* dealing with. It was inconsiderate, and I'm sorry."

That was the foremost concern that had been tearing Grace up as she'd showered. She understood all too well the struggle Max faced every day with his addiction and the last thing he needed was her shoving right into his face the fact that he couldn't have a drink.

For a brief moment, he looked like he was going to argue, but he seemed to think better of it. He rubbed a hand across his chin and nodded. "I appreciate that, but it's okay."

"No, it's not. I wasn't a good friend to you last night. You deserve better and I promise I won't do it again." He opened his mouth to speak, but she continued. "I know you'll say I'm wrong but you know I'm right. Please, just let me grovel?"

He chuckled, his smile relaxed and beautiful. He waved a hand. "Fine. Grovel away."

She pushed her hands into the pockets of her shorts. Max watched her for a quiet, comfortable moment before he took two steps closer. Grace's heart stuttered. It was doing that more and more frequently around him and she couldn't decide whether it was amazing or terrifying.

"I have to admit," he said, his voice low and gravelly. It was his touching-each-other's-fun-parts voice and it immediately did crazy things to her body. Her blood seemed to heat at the same time her organs squeezed lusciously. "Seeing you spread out on the bed in nothing but lace is an image that will live with me for a long time." His eyes lingered down her body while he pressed his tongue to the back of his top teeth. She wanted to know what his tongue tasted like. "You looked hot as fuck, girl."

Her words floated on a slow breath. "I'm glad you liked it."

"I did."

"Maybe I can do it for you again sometime."

He smirked. "Promise?"

"Promise."

"How about when we get back home?"

The way the word "home" struck Grace's chest was altogether too wonderful. "I'm sure I could arrange something."

He smiled wolfishly. "Outstanding. Now, please excuse me. I have to take *another* very cold shower."

She watched him walk away, grumbling to himself about hypothermia, his back muscled, the tattoo exquisite and wet with sweat, making her throat even drier. The bathroom door shut and she heard the water turn on. She fell backward onto the bed and closed her eyes wondering what it would be like to join him in there. The anxiety that rose at the thought was minuscule in comparison to how it had been, but she remained where she was. She knew that she was ready to do more things with Max, not least of all because the electric tension between them was gathering enough voltage to power a small city.

Nevertheless, Grace also knew that her initial friendly intentions toward him were very slowly morphing into something else entirely. Something larger, scarier, something she'd promised herself, promised *him* that she wouldn't allow. It sat silent yet growing in a small cavity in her chest, next to the hope of Max one day maybe feeling the same way.

She placed her hands on her face and breathed, knowing deep down that that was never going to happen. Shit, she was in trouble.

• • • •

"Dude, I can't do this anymore. Can I come and stay with you? Please?"

Max snorted down the phone in reply, lying back on his bed at the boardinghouse while flicking through the channels on the wall-mounted TV. Carter had been whining for the last ten minutes about Kat and their damned wedding. Apparently, Kat's incessant planning and organizing was slowly driving Carter beyond distraction.

"I love her," Carter added. "Truly. I do, but I can't cope with any more talk of being measured for a suit—which you still need to have done, by the way, don't think you can escape this just because your ass isn't here—flowers, and favors. Favors, Max! I didn't even know what a fucking wedding favor is! Do you? I'll tell you: it's a gift you give to the guests. A gift! I mean, why the fuck am *I* giving gifts to people who attend *my* wedding? Where's the fucking sense in that? It's like, yay, you came, here's a twenty-dollar gift for your troubles." There was a thump as though he'd dropped down onto something and he sighed loudly. "I want it to be perfect and I want her to be happy, but I didn't know that women could be . . . I mean, she's just—"

"A fucking nightmare?"

"Yes!" Carter exploded. "Shit!"

Max swiped at the wet paint on his sweatpants. "Should have stayed single, man."

"Right? What the hell was I thinking?" He quieted. "Thing is, when she gets excited about it all . . . man, her face—it's just . . . makes it all worth it, ya know?"

"I'm sure it'll be great."

"Yeah." Carter cleared his throat. "Anyway, enough about that, what's new with you? You have a good July Fourth?"

"Yeah, the cabin was awesome."

"I bet it was. It's been too long since we've made a trip up there. Everyone good? Your uncle okay?"

"He's really great. Still telling tales about me."

"Lemme guess, the pesky front-fastener bra?"

"Asshole."

Carter's laughter grew louder.

Max grinned. "I had a good time."

"Yeah, you sound chill."

Max exhaled. He wasn't too sure he agreed with his friend on that front. The trip to the lake *had* been great, of course, it always was, but his stress levels weren't as low as they probably should have been after four days of doing pretty much nothing.

"Uh-oh," Carter murmured. "That doesn't sound good." There was a beat of silence between the two men, the phone line buzzing with dead air. "You, um, you wanna talk about it?"

Max made a grunting, choking-type noise in response and threw the TV remote to his side, paying no attention to the people on the screen.

"You've spoken to Tate?" Carter prodded. "Or Elliot? Max, if you need something—"

"Carter, I'm fine. Honestly," Max interrupted, his voice softened by his friend's concern. "Actually, it's nothing to do with any of that."

"Huh. Okay. So what's up?"

Max frowned trying to find a simple answer to a complicated question, but the only one he could come up with on the spot was Grace. Max wasn't really sure if he wanted to talk to Carter about Grace because, frankly, he didn't really know what there was to say and, besides, he didn't want Carter to get the wrong impression.

Max's interactions with Grace over Fourth of July had been great, but, admittedly, had also left his head in a bit of a spin. And despite their returning from the cabin three days ago and falling back into their normal working and running routine, they had yet to address the huge fucking elephant in the room every time they were alone together: they still hadn't fucked.

He couldn't remember ever having such a dire case of blue balls and he hated that his patience was fraying. Jesus, the girl had been through a shitload of heartache and Max understood her timidity, but Grace's obliviousness to her own attractiveness had him wanting to throw her down on any nearby horizontal surface and make her forget why she was afraid of sex in the first place.

Since she'd tried to seduce him in her sexy red underwear and then proceeded to vomit up several dollars' worth of alcohol, she'd seemingly taken a step back from him. She was still the easygoing, playful Grace whom Max had grown to know, but the caution he'd seen in her eyes the first time they'd met had returned. And, if Max was truly honest with himself, its appearance had hurt. He'd asked her if she was all right, if he'd done something to upset her, to scare her off, but she'd laughed and waved a dismissive hand at his concerns, telling him that she was fine.

Yeah. That shit was right. She *was* fine. Too damned fine.

He rubbed a hand down his face, noticing another brushstroke of blue paint on his palm. Yeah, he'd even started painting again in an effort to curb his salacious thoughts, to try to stave off the cravings he had for Grace, but it wasn't working. His paintings were, as always, frantic and hurried in their creation, his frustration filling the canvases as quickly as he set them up.

Maybe this was why addicts were told not to start any type of relationships when they were first recovering. It would certainly make sense. Max's desire to lose himself in Grace's body was as strong as his need for coke had been when he first entered rehab.

"Shit." He sat up, still holding the phone to his ear. "Look, man, I'm gonna go. I got some stuff to take care of."

Carter huffed. "Fine. You know where I am if you change your mind. You take care, you hear me?"

Max smiled despite himself. "I will. Later, brother."

He ended the call and threw his cell next to the remote before he changed into a clean pair of shorts, grabbed his Vans, and yanked them onto his feet. He slipped his wallet into his pocket, collected his rental keys, and lifted the painting that had been propped up against his room wall for a number of weeks, hoping it was the icebreaker he and Grace needed.

As she always did, Grace opened the door to her house with a beaming smile. The sound of Marvin Gaye's "Got to Give It Up" was playing in the background. How ironic.

Max smiled back, fidgeting and unexpectedly nervous. "Hey." His eyes traveled down her strapless blue sundress to her bare feet. He smirked at the blue polish on her toes.

"Were we supposed to be meeting for a run today?" She frowned. "I thought you had to work with Vince."

"No. I mean, yeah, I did work," Max replied, flustered. "We finished early so, I, um, I wanted to bring you this." He held up the painting she'd commented on the day she'd brought pizza to his room; the day she'd let him see her naked chest, suck on her nipples, and—

"Really?" she exclaimed, her eyes wide and excited. "I can have this?"

Max shrugged, handing it to her. "Sure. I said so, didn't I?"

Grace grinned. "Thank you. It's wonderful." She spent a moment looking at the canvas of gold, browns, and caramels, and a soft look of something that made Max's stomach clench flittered across her face. "I know exactly where it'll look amazing." She glanced up and tilted her head toward the interior of the house. "I have to be at the bar in a few hours, but you wanna come in? I've just made some lemonade."

Max took a deep breath and nodded. "Sounds good."

The house was truly fantastic now that Grace had all her furniture. Her photographer's eye made sure that all the deco was tasteful and she'd utilized the space perfectly. Max took a moment to appreciate the soft colors of green and cream in which she'd painted the sitting room, and the deep brown leather sofa and light wood coffee table in the center of it. A green rug lay on the floor by a large bookcase of the same beech-wood tones while the walls were punctuated with sepia photographs that Max assumed Grace had taken, leading up the bare wood stairs to the upper level. The July sunshine filled the space through the French windows, which Grace had propped open, bringing the natural colors of the surrounding forest into her home.

He noticed a canvas photograph of two kids on a beach, a boy and a girl—a teenage Grace—neither of them older than sixteen, arms around each other, the braces on the boy's teeth clear to see, his legs, like his body, long and gangly.

"My brother. He looks entirely different now. He took a long time to grow into himself."

"He's younger than you?" Max asked.

"Yeah, a year, but he's the one who looks after me." She looked over the other photographs in the room. "I need to get some recent photos of him, but he's about as fond of having his picture taken as you are."

Max's gaze moved to another photograph, this one in a wooden frame. It was black-and-white and appeared sun damaged, leaving the image faded in parts. A tall black man with an exceptionally cool Afro, dressed in tight-fitted shirt and jeans, stood with his arm around a striking dark-haired white woman whose smile was as big as the one Max saw on Grace's face when she laughed.

"Mom and Dad," she said softly, looking fondly at the picture. "Mom was from Preston County. She met dad in DC. They were together for twenty years before he passed away. Mom managed ten years without him." She glanced up at Max. "Heart disease." She looked back at the picture. "Kai and I always believed she died of a broken heart."

"She's beautiful," Max murmured.

"Yeah, she was."

Max followed Grace into the kitchen, where she handed him a cold glass of lemonade.

"Mom's recipe. Homemade," she said with a wink.

"I should hope so," Max replied, taking a long sip. The silence stretched out between them, fizzing and sparking like it always did when they were alone. Max wondered fleetingly if that was why Grace had retreated from him. It was certainly an odd feeling. He leaned a hip against the kitchen counter, watching her as she pretended to wipe condensation off her glass. "So," he began, placing his glass down. "I was thinking maybe we could talk."

Her eyes snapped to his, worry creasing their edges. "Talk?"

Max swallowed and cleared his throat. "I wanted to make sure that everything was still okay. You know, with us." He gestured with a finger between them.

Grace blinked. "Us?"

"Yeah." He exhaled and dropped his shoulders. "I mean, you seem . . . different and— We're good, right?"

Grace shook her head gently from side to side. "Why on earth would you think we weren't?" She didn't give him a chance to answer. "You've been nothing but amazing, Max. You've been a good friend." She licked her lips. "A *great* friend."

A smile tugged at the corners of Max's mouth. Grace put her glass next to his and moved closer, her gaze on her fingers as they danced along the side of the counter. "I know I've been a little distant since the cabin. And I'm sorry. I was just so damned mortified by what happened the night we went out that I didn't know whether you wanted anything more to happen or how to even broach the subject."

Max nudged her foot with his own. "Hey, I told you. You can talk to me about anything." He watched her shoulders relax. "And, seriously, woman, I still want the 'anything more' to happen."

"Yeah?"

Max rolled his eyes. "Pfft, shut up."

Grace's heavy expression lifted. "Even though I vomited and made a spectacle of myself?"

"Even then. And trust me, if you wear underwear like that every time you vomit, I'd absolutely be okay with that. Gives me something nice to look at while I'm holding your hair back, right?"

They both laughed.

"Okay," Grace said on a long breath. She regarded him for a moment. "Okay."

Max felt the anxiety he'd been harboring about their conversation drift away on the breeze whispering through the house. "So the place looks awesome." He pointed to a part of the kitchen wall that he'd rebuilt and plastered. "Especially that bit. That part's my favorite."

Grace sipped her drink before almost choking on it in excitement. "Oh, hey! I need to show you something." Putting her empty glass in the sink, she grabbed Max's wrist and pulled him toward the stairs. "I forgot to tell you!"

Max chuckled as he followed her up to the first level of the house. She released him and quickly closed a door that was slightly ajar, looking embarrassed. Max looked at her in question. "Dead bodies?"

"Not quite. My darkroom. I've been working on the photographs for my show."

"Yeah?" Max asked excitedly. "The ones of me? Can I see?"

Grace shook her head firmly. "Not yet. The collection's not finished. I have something better to show you." She led him down the corridor to the room Max knew to be her bedroom.

Better indeed.

She pushed the door open, stepped into the room, and opened her arms wide. "Ta-da!"

The last time Max had seen her bedroom, when he'd been hauling all the heavy-ass furniture around for her, Grace's place of sleep had been a blowup mattress on the floor. Now in its place was a wrought-iron framed bed, decorated in a white comforter and stacks of pillows. The fucking thing was huge.

"Wow," he murmured, stepping closer.

"Right? Isn't it awesome?" Grace bounced around the bed to the other side and clambered onto it. She lay down and patted the space next to her. "Here. Try it."

Seeing her on her back all bare arms and legs was a real test of Max's resolve. He cocked his head to the side and lifted a curious eyebrow.

"Oh, stop," she chastised with a smirk. "I just want you to feel it."

Max barked a laugh. "Shit, it's been a long time since I've heard a woman say that to me."

He toed off his shoes and eyed her suspiciously. He pointed to the bed. "Seriously, though, are you propositioning me? Because, I'll be honest, I'm totally fucking fine with that."

"Just shush and lie down."

Relaxing, Max sat down on the bed before swinging his legs onto it. He launched a couple of pillows down to the foot of it so they didn't smother him to death and adjusted himself into a comfortable position: on his back, his hands laced on his stomach. "Damn," he muttered, shuffling a little. "This shit *is* comfortable."

"I told you," Grace replied, her words laced with smugness.

Max turned his head to watch her. "I love it," she added, closing her eyes. "I've never had a huge bed all to myself before."

"Really?"

"Really. I can starfish and no one can stop me."

She moved her arm outward, showing Max how she could starfish like it was her job. Sure enough, even with him next to her in the monster bed, she had room to spread out. Max copied her as she moved her arms and legs, as if they were making snow angels on the duvet, and her hand touched his. They both paused. Grace glanced over at him and gently rubbed Max's pinkie with her own.

The contact made the ball of desire in his belly twist and the muscle in his jaw tic as he clenched his teeth together. He exhaled heavily and shuffled some more into the ultracomfy bedding, trying to ignore the way the atmosphere around them changed, sharpened, and how it caused his pulse to thunder through his body.

"So I have a question," Grace whispered.

"Shoot."

She moved closer, rolling slowly onto her side, her breath warm on his cheek. "What if I was?"

His eyes slid over to hers, though her focus was on his chest. She watched, seemingly fascinated as it lifted and dropped with the heavy breaths he was taking. "What if you was what?"

Their eyes met gradually and Max's lungs squeezed. "What if I was . . ." She lifted a shoulder. "Propositioning you?"

He stared at her for a beat, dragging air into lungs that were now apparently finding it really fucking hard to do their job. "You teasing me again?" The words sounded ever so slightly bitter off his tongue, which wasn't Max's intention, but, shit, he couldn't cope with another game of look but don't touch. He wanted to touch; he wanted to touch her everywhere.

Grace lifted onto her forearm so that she was above him. "No," she whispered with a gentle shake of her head. "I'm not teasing."

22

It was as though a vacuum pulled all the air from the room as she spoke. Wordless, Max pushed his head back into the pillows beneath it, making sure that he could see all of her face, trying to detect any hint of dishonesty. As was always the way with Grace, he found none. His gaze traveled over her, starting with her bright eyes, which were always truthful, to her mouth so plump and eager, down to her neck and her fucking awesome chest. "You sure?"

"When you look at me like that?" she breathed. "Yes, I'm sure."

"How am I looking at you?"

"Like you want me."

"I do."

She moved gradually, sitting up. "I know." Max made to sit up with her, but her small hand on his chest pushed him back down. "Stay."

All Max could do was nod. He watched her hand move over his chest and down to his stomach, slow and careful until it reached the hem of his T-shirt. She pulled it up, exposing his skin, which she touched reverently. This was okay, Max thought, breathing deeply. He was prepared for this. She'd done this before.

What she hadn't done before, however, was place those fucking stupendous lips against his stomach and kiss him. Fuck, her mouth was so damned soft. He released a low grunt when she did it again and her mouth moved across his clenched muscles, around his belly button, and up toward his chest, pushing his T-shirt up the farther she went.

Max lifted a little from the bed, pulling the damned thing over his head, and dropped it to the floor. Carefully, with his fingers, he pushed her hair back, not holding her—knowing her aversion to being restrained in any way—but keeping it back from her face. He wanted to see her, see her explore his body. He wanted to capture every single moment because, fuck, he'd never seen anything as erotic as Grace taking control. He fisted the bedsheets with his free hand, clenching and releasing, instead of succumbing to the overwhelming need he had to grab her, throw her down, and have his way with her.

As if reading his mind, she hummed with a smile into his skin and Jesus fucking *Christ* when her tongue came out to taste his nipple, Max almost leaped from the bed.

"You taste good," she said into his chest, her fingers moving through the hair that speckled it. She sighed. "I want to taste you all over."

"Goddamn," Max uttered, grimacing at his uncomfortable hard-on. His hips flexed with the need for any type of friction. "Do what you want," he urged. "Please. Anything."

She glanced down at his predicament. "Can I . . . would it be okay if I undressed you?"

Max scoffed and quickly pushed the button through the hole on his shorts, eager to get her started. "Grace. Don't ask." He opened his arms wide, offering himself to her white-hot stare. "Just touch."

She kneeled up and clasped the fly zipper, pulling it down too fucking slowly. Max lifted his hips and pushed his fingers into the waistband at his lower back, helping her pull the godforsaken things down his thighs. He kicked them off his feet, leaving him in nothing but his boxer briefs, tented with his want. Max bit his lip when her finger traced the outline of him through his underwear.

"You're so hard," she murmured.

"You have no fucking idea," he replied, holding back an incredulous laugh. "Take them off me."

For a split second, Max saw her waver, he saw anxiety and doubt, and his stomach dropped. He opened his mouth to reassure her, to tell her that, despite him and his cock wanting nothing more than to have her bouncing all over it, it was okay, that they didn't have to do anything, that they'd take it slow, but, God bless her, he didn't get the chance.

Without preamble, Grace pushed her small fingers into the elastic of his underwear and pulled. Max didn't hesitate. He lifted up, allowing her to rid him of them, and kicked them off his feet to the end of the bed.

Naked and hard as hell, Max lay back and allowed Grace to stare at him.

Her green gaze wandered from the tip of his toes to the crown of his head and back again, roaming over his cock in such a way that Max was pretty certain he could have come from that particular look alone.

"You're . . . exquisite," she whispered, reaching out a hand to caress his erection. He growled at the sensation of someone other than himself touching—it had been too fucking long—the gentle stroke, the throb that craved more, harder, firmer.

He swallowed back a moan when she gripped him and slid her hand up and down, cautious yet determined. "What the hell's wrong with this picture?"

With her eyes still on his dick in her hand she replied, "Absolutely nothing."

He laughed gently, bringing her eyes back to his. "Grace." He lifted a hand and stroked her thigh. "I'm naked and you're not." She glanced down at herself as though surprised by the fact. "Let me see you," he urged. "You're in control here, Grace. I'll do whatever you want, but I want to see you." He squeezed her leg. Still on her knees, she released him, appearing to consider him carefully. "I've got you," he murmured. "Trust me."

She took a deep breath and lifted her dress up and over her

head, leaving her in a pair of black panties and nothing else. Her hair fell down her shoulders and back and her dark skin was so fucking beautiful in the soft light that filtered through the white lace, which hung at her bedroom window. Her scars—her tiger stripes, as Max had come to call them—moved like ripples on a pond as she discarded her dress to the floor.

"Perfect," he said softly when he saw her fidget under his appreciative stare. Max couldn't help but touch. He reached out and cupped her tits, loving their weight in his hands and the pebbling of her nipples against his palms. "Fuck, yeah."

"What do you want?" Grace gasped, arching her back and pushing more of herself into his grasp.

"Whatever *you* fucking want," he replied before licking her stomach.

"Max, tell me." The slight pleading in her voice brought Max's head up. "I want to know. Please?"

Max moved back, resting his weight on his elbow. He rubbed a hand through his hair as a barrage of filthy, hot, and sweaty images assaulted his mind. He chuckled nervously. "Grace, this is all on you. I don't think—"

"Max," she interrupted, placing her hand back on his cock.

He swallowed and closed his eyes as he spoke. "I want you to ride my face. I want you to come all over my mouth because I'm desperate to taste you. Then I want you to do the same to my cock, because I don't think I can wait another second not being inside of you."

Max opened his eyes when a low moan echoed around him.

"Jesus, O'Hare," Grace gasped. "You don't mess around, do you?"

"You mean . . . you like the sound of that?"

She bit her lip, dropped down next to him, and pushed her underwear off. Max kept his eyes on hers, even though he was nearly turning himself inside out with the need to see her fully naked. They breathed together, watching the other tenderly before Max spoke.

"You can get on whenever you're ready," he said. A burst of nervous laughter erupted from her, relaxing Max further. He knew he had to assure her, make her comfortable, but he continued to find himself fumbling. Fuck it, he was like a damned virgin, jumpy and about ready to come at the mere hint of a pair of spread legs.

"Stop," Grace said softly, placing a hand over his racing heart. "Stop overthinking it. I'm okay." She leaned over then, placing a soft, chaste kiss on his cheek. "I'm supposed to be the intimacy nutcase here, not you."

Max lay back. "In that case, have at me."

She lifted gradually, every movement steady, every shift of her body measured. She was fucking breathtaking to look at. She gripped the wrought-iron headboard and glanced at Max, her brow furrowing. She opened her mouth to speak.

"Don't," Max said quietly. "Please. You're fine. You look incredible." She raised her leg and dropped down so that she was straddling his chest and Max got a fucking epic view of every part of her, bare and perfect. He ran his palms up her thighs, to her waist, and back again, keeping his touch light so as not to panic her. "Come here. Let me taste."

Grace moved over him and, when his lips finally met the ones between her legs, Max was sure he saw fucking stars, and, oh, holy fuck, she was wet. Soaked. He groaned. Unable to be patient, his tongue slid against her clit, garnering from her a squeal of gibberish and a jump of surprise.

"Max! I— Oh."

Grace's hips swiveled and lifted, as though the feeling was too much, but Max held her legs softly, coaxing her body to ease against him, humming against her flesh. "It's okay. I've got you."

Her taste was fucking exquisite, creamy, and sour in all the right ways. Max hummed against her swollen clit and lathered every inch of her with his mouth. Grace writhed and moaned loudly. His rapid and willing tongue finally disappeared inside her, becoming a part of her, pulsing into her tightness with every surge and dip of her hips.

Shit, she smelled fantastic, too; the subtle hint of cocoa butter, along with the scent of her when they ran, set him alight. A deep sound from her throat came again when Max kissed her skin, letting his eager tongue and lips glide over her. He teased her clit between his lips, gently grazing her with his teeth, causing her to call out.

While his mouth tasted, his hands moved slowly across her stomach to the hips that were moving in figures of eight, driving him fucking insane. He gripped them gently and pushed his mouth firmly against her. An exquisite groan escaped her, forcing Max to do it again. He opened his eyes to see that her head had fallen back, her black hair spilling down her back, tickling his stomach when he breathed in. Max brought his hand up and stroked Grace's neck, feeling the thrum of her pulse under his gentle fingertips. She panted his name, spurring his tongue on until she was riding his face just as he'd hoped, thrusting and shuddering above him.

Grace's hand appeared suddenly, grabbing his hair and pushing his face harder against her. The fact that she wanted him this way, that she was enjoying it and wanted more, made Max's cock twitch between his legs.

Jesus.

"I'm— Oh, God!"

Fuck, Max had almost forgotten what it was like to hear a woman beg, plead, come on him, because of him. He sucked and licked, dipping his tongue into her again, softly at first, gauging her reaction, before he pushed it harder, feeling her body give to him, open up to him, welcome him with open fucking arms. His own body pulsed and wept as he feasted, his pulse thundered in his ears, and, when Grace began to cry out, he wished to all hell that he could see her face clearly as she came.

"I can't—it's . . . Yes, oh. Yes!" she chanted, bucking and crying out as she exploded on his lips.

He pushed his face farther into her, crying out for more of the wetness that drenched his mouth and chin. She laced her fingers together at the back of his head and held him to her body.

"Fuck," he mumbled into her flesh, while his eyes rolled back into his skull.

As the pulse of her orgasm resonated through his tongue, he lapped up everything she gave. It was fucking glorious. The aroma of her and the feel of her sopping skin was almost enough for Max to lose his damned mind. Grace panted and cursed softly until, unable to take any more, she moved back off his face, now slick with her orgasm, and slid, somewhat awkwardly, to her side of the bed.

Max blew out a long breath, licked his lips, and wiped the back of his hand across his face. Her smell was all around him and he allowed himself a couple of quiet heavy-breathing-filled moments to bask in it. His cock thrummed and jerked, aching for relief, but Max resisted touching, waiting for Grace to say or do something. He looked over to see her face covered in her hair. The parts of her that he could see through it showed a serene smile, which pulled his mouth into one of its own.

"You all right?" he asked quietly.

She nodded, still smiling.

"You coherent?" She shook her head, making Max laugh. "Then my work here is done."

When she neither moved nor spoke, he lifted his upper body from the bed and reached for his clothes and underwear, which were stuffed between the pillows he'd thrown. Once again, he was stopped by Grace's hand on his arm.

"Where you going?" she asked, her voice sexily hoarse from her cries despite her expression, which, once she'd brushed back her hair, Max could only describe as confused and maybe a little hurt.

"Hey, I'm not running out on you." He glanced down at himself. "I was, um, going to clean up, then head home to take care of this." He waved a hand at his twitching crotch. He smiled. "I just thought you'd want to—"

"I want to make you come, Max. I want to try what you said, you know— Can I?"

Well, couldn't he just leap with joy hearing those fucking words?

"But . . ." Max cleared his throat, lying back. "Not that I'm not fucking ecstatic by the mere idea of you being my own personal cowgirl, but are you sure?"

Grace cocked an unimpressed eyebrow and pursed her lips. "Max, you just gave me the first orgasm I've had with another person in the room in a very long time. You've helped me get over the hurdle of years of self-consciousness and fear by"—she looked at his mouth, her eyes dilating further—"doing that *amazing* thing with your tongue. I mean, how the hell did you do that with the . . . you know, the way you . . ."

Pride rushed through him at the thought of his truly making her feel good and finding her just about the most adorable thing ever.

She gathered herself, taking a deep breath. "Please, Max. I want to repay the favor. Will you let me?"

Max held up his hands. "Okay. Okay," he deadpanned. "I suppose I can manage that." He laughed when she shoved him playfully, before lowering his voice and staring at the space between her legs. "I guess I'll just have to let you ride my cock."

She licked her lips. "Do you have . . . something?"

"In my wallet." Max motioned toward his shorts and watched as Grace leaned over him to grab them. Unable to help himself, Max sat up and, holding her by her thighs, nibbled his way across her ass cheeks.

Grace startled. "What the—?"

"Fuck, your ass is insane," he moaned, licking and biting gently.

"*You're* insane," she teased lightly, shooing him away and sitting back up. She held the foil packet out to Max and watched as he tore it open. She noticed his pointed look as he held the latex above his cock. "I'm fine," she murmured, her face soft and gorgeous, the determination faltering ever so slightly. "I want to at least try."

Max exhaled. "We stop immediately if you're not happy doing this, you got me?" Her gaze stayed on his hands as he rolled on the condom. "You're in charge. We go as fast or as slow as you want."

She nodded and moved toward him, straddling his thighs, and fingering his balls as if she'd never seen a pair before. Not that Max minded. Christ, if she kept going they'd have no need to go any further. He'd bust a nut right then.

"Gracie," he whispered.

"I love it when you call me that." She glanced up at him through her lashes. "Can you . . . can you help me—"

"Whatever you need," he preempted, holding a hand out, which she took. He squeezed her fingers between his as she lifted and wrapped her other hand around his cock, guiding him to her. Max's chest burned as he held his breath, watching. The tip of him swiped over her gently, pulling a husky moan from them both. Their eyes met and Max's breath shook from him.

"I've got you," he murmured, and lifted his hips ever so slightly, pushing against where he was desperate to be.

"I know." Grace lifted her face toward the ceiling, eyes closed, bottom lip between her teeth as she released his cock and allowed her weight to pull her down onto it. Max groaned, watching himself disappear into her, her body enveloping every inch of him, gripping him so fucking tightly he could barely stand it. Fuck, how long had it been? She sat on him, quiet and breathing steadily, adjusting herself with minute shifts of her hips that shot blazing heat through every inch of Max's body.

"Jesus," he managed through gritted teeth, his eyebrows meeting above his nose as he grimaced. "Are you okay?"

"Mmhm," she hummed in response. "Max, it . . . you feel amazing."

Max clenched his eyes shut, gripping her with one hand and the bedsheets with the other. "Move," he pleaded. "For the love of God, please move."

Max felt her body trembling above him before she slowly moved her hips in a way that lifted her from him. He grunted when he saw the light from the window glint off the wetness Grace's body had left on the condom. She didn't lift too far before she dropped back down, patient and, Max had to admit, insanely hot. Her body embraced his, squeezing him as though it was fucking delighted to have him there. She gasped when he tilted his hips at the same time she sank down, pushing even farther into her.

"That's it," he murmured, his brow breaking out in a sweat with the effort it took not to slam up faster. "You feel so good."

"Yes," she gasped. "God. I'd forgotten, I— Oh, you fill me."

"Fuck, Gracie," Max replied, gritting his teeth at the same time he thrust gently. "Keep going."

Max breathed deeply out his nose as she found her rhythm, rotating her hips, lifting and dropping. She fucked him slowly, but Max couldn't have cared less. Watching her take her pleasure from him was more than enough to have his orgasm gripping his stomach and tightening his thighs. She released his hand and placed her palms on his chest, pushing against him as she increased her speed. Max's grip immediately found her hips. Their eyes met for a split second, his seeking out her permission to hold her that way. She smiled her consent—she was fine, her gaze whispered—and groaned when the slap of their flesh meeting echoed around the room.

He pressed his head back into the pillow, elongating his neck, closing his eyes, and allowed his body to accept the pleasure Grace was conjuring from him. "Tell me you've thought about this," he grunted.

"Yes," she answered. "So much."

"Tell me," he repeated, arching his back as she dropped onto him again. "How?"

"At the cottage on the tree trunk, at the bar where people can hear us, see us."

"Fuck yes," Max replied, heat flashing through him at the mere thought of people hearing her scream his name.

"In the shower," she continued, moving faster. "In my kitchen on the countertop, on my sofa, against the window so everyone can see what you do to me. In your truck while you drive."

"Goddamn," Max gasped, struck dumb by the words leaving Grace's panting, wet mouth. Her fingernails pinched his stomach, ripping a moan from his chest and sending his hips up quickly.

"More," Grace whimpered. "Please more."

Max complied, pushing harder, digging his heels into the duvet and driving his cock deeper, faster, his knees pressing into her perfect ass, until the bed began to creak and the room grew hot, stifled with their fucking and the sounds that erupted from them with little warning. Max lost himself in Grace's heat, her soaked flesh, her grabby hands, and her calls out for more. He watched her unfurl before him, her timid, quiet exterior crashing around them on the bed, revealing a tigress, a sexual creature incapable of being anything but wild and wanton. She was a fucking vision. She rode him and pulled from him every ounce of exquisite feeling he thought himself able to possess.

His hands moved to her waist as he thrust deeper, eliciting a scream from the depths of Grace's throat.

"Yeah?" he grunted. "Am I hitting it right? Right there, Gracie?"

"Shit," she exclaimed, her head bobbing, her neck unable to hold it up as Max fucked her.

With his eyes fixed on hers, Max drove up. Again. Again. Thrust. Pause. Thrust. Pause.

Christ, she felt so fucking good. She enveloped him like a second skin, snug, perfect, slick, and warm. He pushed farther into her, making her breath catch.

Again. Again.

Feeling his body start to take over, Max gripped Grace's hips tighter. He held on, feeling the muscles in his forearms and shoulders pull and cord with every thrust. She moaned again as her knees squeezed his sides. With a deep moan and a series of strong slaps of his thighs against her ass, Max watched Grace above him, bouncing gloriously.

"Don't stop," he ordered before his throat began to bark out incomprehensible sounds and words.

He held her. He held her so tightly, as she moved. But she never panicked, she never told him not to. She took every thrust, every shove of his body into hers. She looked sensational with her head thrown back, neck elongated, and her tits begging for his lips. Unable to resist any longer, Max sat up with a moan and sucked her hard nipple into his mouth, and hummed into her soft skin when she bucked against him.

Grace cried out. "More."

He gave her more. She wrapped her arms around his neck, as she wound her pelvis in a luscious circle that nearly made him lose his damned mind.

"Close," he croaked as his hips started to piston upward, lifting her knees from the mattress. His orgasm was building, deep in his balls, stretching to his stomach.

Feeling all his energy start to push down into his groin, Max fell back onto the pillows, watching in breathless wonder as Grace continued to pull it from him. She lifted and fell, she demanded and begged, she swiveled and clenched, she thrust and grasped until, with a furious roar, Max exploded into her.

His back arched and his neck corded with its strength. "Holy fuck!"

Bright lights blinded him, as his body twitched and shivered.

Grace continued to ride him, moaning as his cock twitched inside her, relief seizing Max from his head to his feet, as waves of euphoria crashed over him until he couldn't take it. He held Grace fast, stilling her movements, moaning at her to please, God, stop. The small part of his brain that remained in his skull and wasn't splattered on the ceiling like the rest of it grimaced when he realized Grace hadn't come again.

Her small body eventually collapsed onto his chest, and he immediately felt her pulse as it raced under the delicately soft skin of her spine. Max's limp arms held her, spent and breathing heavily. He was exhausted, mentally and physically, and his eyes closed briefly of their own volition, despite his attempts at keeping them open.

Still panting and with his heart doing laps behind his ribs, he patted her back gently. "Can you—? I need to get rid of this."

Sweaty and glorious, Grace placed her hands on his chest and lifted her body slowly. Max gripped the base of the condom, hissing at the friction, and sat up as she plopped down at his side. "I'll be back in a minute."

Washed up, buck-ass naked, and feeling pretty damned great, Max strolled back into the bedroom to find Grace sitting cross-legged in the middle of the bed wearing a large black T-shirt that covered every fantastic inch of her. "Spoil sport," he teased, smiling. He kneeled beside her and moved his hand between her legs, seeking out her clit. Grace's fingers on his wrist made him pause.

"It's all right," she whispered, her smile dopey and gorgeous. "Honestly."

Max's hand dropped to the bed with a thump. He sighed and reached for his underwear. "If you're sure," he muttered, pulling on his boxer briefs, glancing at her surreptitiously for any sign of freak-out or regret. To his relief, he saw none.

She watched him as he dressed. "You're superthorough, huh?" Max looked at her questioningly. She looked pointedly toward the bathroom. The condom.

"Yeah, well," he replied, sitting down to put on his shorts. "We don't want any accidents. Believe me, they happen."

"Christopher was an accident?"

Max swallowed at the sound of his son's name. "He wasn't planned."

"But you and Lizzie, you both wanted him, right?"

Max paused, keeping his eyes on the floor. "Yes. Yes, we both wanted him very much."

"But you'd never consider having kids again?" Grace's voice was soft. "Ever?"

Max yanked on his shorts, leaving them undone, and adjusted himself on the bed, sitting with his back against the headboard. "I don't know," he answered honestly, his fingers trailing a path through his hair. "I . . . I couldn't go through that again." His heart twisted in his chest. "Seeing the person you love shatter like that."

Grace moved closer, the smell of their sex wafting around them as the blankets moved, conjuring an interested pulse from Max's cock despite the topic of conversation. "What happened with Christopher was tragic, Max, but it's also rare." She squeezed his hand. "You shouldn't close yourself off to the possibility—"

"Look," Max bristled, his just-got-laid buzz changing into something darker, something that lay dormant only because his meds and his therapy kept it so. He pulled his hand away. "I know what you're saying but those things that women want—love, babies, a future—I don't have the ability to provide those." His voice was sharp, making Grace flinch. He paused and exhaled. "I did. Once. But they were lost a long time ago and they're not ever coming back."

He kept his eyes on the bed covers, praying to all shit that, now that they'd slept together, Grace wouldn't suddenly start to want more. From the cavity in his chest that echoed with her question about kids, Max knew there was no way he could give her or any other woman anything other than his body. He glanced up, the expression on Grace's face sad but somehow understanding.

"Well, who knows," she said softly. "Maybe they'll come back when you least expect it."

Max didn't believe that for a second but he gave her a small smile all the same. "I'd better go."

Grace blinked. "You're free to stay. I'm sorry. I didn't mean to bring up—"

"Hey, it's all right," Max interrupted, standing from the bed. "Honestly." He bent down and placed a soft kiss on her cheek. He stood back. "Are you really okay? Was I . . . was it good?" He wasn't looking to have his ego stroked. He simply wanted to make sure she'd enjoyed it and that the demons he knew she carried weren't hounding her behind that stunning smile.

That smile grew and her eyes lightened, calming Max's anxiety. "Yes. I'm . . . great. You— it was . . . perfect."

"Good." He pulled on his T-shirt.

"Thank you, Max. Really. Thank you."

"It was my pleasure. You were wonderful." He grabbed his Vans from the floor and cleared his throat. "I'll see you later."

Pushing the guilt that skittered across his neck down into the darkest parts of him, Max left Grace sitting on her bed. He was unable to truly breathe until he pushed through her front door, staggering into the blazing sunshine.

23

"Holy shit! Look at you!"

Grace smiled at the loud, excited voice that echoed around her brother's club.

"You're a sight for sore eyes, baby girl."

Grace watched Sienna Kelly, Kai's assistant bar manager, bound across the dance floor from the main entrance of the club, her tight Afro bouncing as she went. The deep red lipstick that covered her insane lips was striking and indescribably sexy against her ebony skin, while her outfit was, as always, tight and left little to the imagination. She was, in her own words, a workout maniac, and it showed. Her body was incredible. Grace opened her arms and accepted Sienna's enthusiastic hug, laughing as Sienna kissed her cheek.

"You look beautiful," Sienna exclaimed, holding Grace at arm's length. "Why the hell has it been so long since I've seen you?"

"Because one of us has been off exploring the world," Grace replied. "How was Europe?"

"Oh my God, girl," Sienna replied. "It was unbelievable." She turned and leaned her hip against the fridge underneath the bar. "Paris, Rome, London, it was all fabulous. I didn't want to come back."

"I don't blame you! Paris sure beats the hell out of Washington, DC."

Sienna reached for a bottle of Corona and snapped off the top, holding it out to Grace. "Let me tell you, if it wasn't for your asshole of a brother, I'd still be there."

Grace smiled at the affection she heard in Sienna's voice despite her language. Grace was fairly certain that Sienna and Kai had been involved at some stage and that Sienna, contrary to outward appearances, was a little bit smitten. Grace knew that her brother could do a damn sight worse. Sienna was vivacious and sharp-tongued, but she was the most loyal and trustworthy person Grace knew besides Kai. Underneath the banter and sniping, the two of them were perfect for one another.

"So tell me about you," Sienna continued, sipping from her own Corona. "How's West Virginia? Kai told me you bought a house."

Grace nodded and sipped her drink. "It's great. The house is amazing. I'm working and I've made some really nice friends. I feel safe there."

"That's awesome," Sienna said. "I'm so proud of you." She hugged Grace again. "So what brings you here?"

"I have a therapist appointment tomorrow and Kai said he was understaffed." Grace kicked at the box of beer bottles she'd been emptying into the fridge. "I thought I'd lend a hand."

It was kind of the truth. Grace did have an appointment with her therapist and Kai *was* understaffed, but she hadn't really needed to be in DC until tomorrow. Had anyone asked, Grace would have said she was there because Holly didn't need her at Whiskey's until the weekend and she wanted to spend time with her brother; the truth was, she was there because she needed space.

Since that afternoon in her bed when the scent and feel of Max's body next to hers had forced away her panic, leaving only desire in its wake; the afternoon she'd taken control, ignored her inhibitions, and had the best sex of her life, she and Max had fooled around twice more. And Lord, what fun it had been. Seeing Max naked beneath her, mouth open, breathless and damp with sweat was now Grace's most favorite thing. He was gorgeously animal in his passion, handling her with such care, yet giving her everything she asked for when she pleaded with him to give it harder, faster.

Never had she seen anything as beautiful as Max when, the second time they'd had sex, she'd ridden him on her couch, her back to his chest, his breath hot on her neck, and his hands firm on her ass, shouting out his curses and coming hard with her. She loved the feel of him, so strong and solid, the way his face creased when he came, and the sound of her name on his lips as he pulsed inside her.

Knowing that she could do for him what he did for her filled her with a profound happiness. Seeing him sated and drowsy, that lopsided smile and those dark, playful eyes focused on her as they moved together, filled her with something more, however, something heavy and hopeful.

As Max would say, she was well and truly fucked, and spending a few days away from him and from the desire that accosted her every time they were in the same room seemed like a wise idea. She couldn't risk Max sensing the way she was starting to feel about him. Was already feeling about him. Jesus, at the mere mention of his having kids in the future he'd paled and run from her. God alone knew what he'd do if he realized she was falling for him. Grace wanted him in her life too much—regardless of the capacity—to jeopardize what they had together. His friendship had become too important, too integral to her day-to-day life.

The quiet times they spent together were as precious as the sexy times. Just yesterday, after she'd watched him come all over her stomach while she lay on the pale green rug in her living room, they'd lain side by side, talking about art, music, and more about her family.

Max, in turn, spoke of his own parents. As she listened, Grace lost herself in his voice and the way his arm brushed against hers when he moved. They'd ordered pizza and sat together, half-naked as they ate it, so comfortable with each other that Grace hadn't even bothered to cover up her scars. There was no point. Besides, the way he looked at her naked body made Grace forget about everything else anyway. Never had she felt so desired, wanted, so beautiful as when Max's gaze was on her.

That had only been twenty-four hours ago and already she'd started to miss him.

"It's fantastic that you're so comfortable with Max," Nina, Grace's therapist, mused the following afternoon. "It really is; you've embraced intimacy again and it's lovely to see you moving forward, taking control back, but these feelings you have . . . they may be detrimental to you both."

This Grace knew. Max was a fragile creature, an addict, he was vulnerable and skittish, but there was no way she was going to stop sleeping with him just because she couldn't keep her emotions in check. She would do it. For him, she *could* do it.

"Grace, these steps you're taking are excellent, it's great news."

"But?"

"But you need to be clear on what it is you're feeling." Nina shifted in her seat. "Tell me, when he walked out after you had sex the first time, how did you feel?"

Grace shrugged, tracing the lip of the coffee cup in her hand with her finger. She thought back to that amazing afternoon. Max's words and his longing for her so clear in his large Hershey's Kiss eyes. His hard body, his skin on her tongue, the way he knew that, without her even saying, she had to be on top so she didn't freak out. The sounds he made, and the crushing need she'd had to smash her lips to his and taste and own every groan and gasp.

"I knew he needed to leave," she answered, her face heating with the memories. "He was very clear on what our relationship would be when we agreed to this. I can't expect hugs and kisses afterward."

"That's what you wanted?"

Not exactly. It had been a very long time since she'd experienced cuddles after sex, so she wasn't expecting it now. Grace would have liked Max to have stayed a little while longer, of course, because seeing him rush out the door, although expected, had been hard. Not that she'd ever tell him. No, instead, the following day, she'd woken Max at the boardinghouse with coffee and a muffin and dragged him out on their run. Normal routine was important for both of them. It was pretty clear that Grace wasn't the only one of them who had the potential to freak out.

"Grace," Nina said softly. "Getting close to Max, being his friend is one thing. Having a sexual relationship and allowing yourself to feel more is something else entirely. My question is, are you really ready and, just as important, is Max?"

Grace sighed, not having an answer. "You're saying I shouldn't allow myself to feel something for him?"

"No, Grace," Nina said, her blue eyes careful behind her red spectacles. "I'm saying I want you to remember that you're both brittle creatures who've been through a lot of trauma. To remember that it isn't *your* job to fix everyone and not everyone wants fixing. I'm saying I want you to prepare yourself for what may happen here."

Her point was unspoken yet clear: he'll break your heart, Grace. But, honestly, Grace couldn't have cared less.

· · ·

"Oh my God," Max complained with a shake of his head as he stood outside the coffee shop. "Did you have to bring *him* with you?"

Tate laughed while crossing the street toward Max and glanced over to Riley at his side.

"Come here, you motherfucker!" Riley called out before, with a loud whoop, he took off at speed.

Max braced himself for the impact, knowing how heavy and solid Riley was. The air in Max's body burst from him in a resounding *oomph* when Riley connected, wrapping him in a huge bear hug and tilting them to the side. Max only just managed to stay on his feet and keep his aviator shades on his face while cursing the bastard up and down.

"I missed you, too, you ugly shit," Riley said with a laugh, ruffling Max's hair.

Max pushed him away with a chuckle and shook Tate's hand. "Good to see you."

"You, too," Tate replied, slowly lifting a suspicious eyebrow. "You look well and . . ." He cocked his head. "Decidedly pleased with yourself."

Riley gasped, not missing a beat. "You got laid?"

Max laughed at the two apparently telepathic brothers standing there like peas in a damn pod with their hugeness and wide, smiling faces. If Riley didn't have his beard and Tate's hair was longer, they'd easily pass for twins.

"Sweet Jesus," Max grumbled, pushing past them. "Can we eat before we start this kind of talk? I'm starved."

"Ha!" Riley exclaimed, following Max through the door. "See, that right there, Tate, is your customary O'Hare blow-off. He's hiding something."

"Or someone," Tate added at his side. Max turned to his sponsor to see him surveying the customers already seated with their drinks and food. "Where's Running Girl?"

"Who's Running Girl?" Riley asked with a grin.

"Her name is Grace, as I recall."

"Nice. She hot?"

"Smokin' hot," Tate answered, biting his lip. He waved toward Max. "These two are 'running partners,' apparently."

Riley scoffed. "Yeah. I've had lots of those."

"I met her when she was trussed up in her gear," Tate continued.

Riley made an obscene noise. "Tight running pants?"

"The tightest."

"Nice ass?"

"Epic. Shapely, you know, tiny waist, wide hips, and these lips that just—"

"Okay!" Max yelled as loud as was appropriate in a coffee shop on a Saturday afternoon. He waved his hands in a large T shape. "Time-out!" The brothers smiled at him in satisfaction, arms crossed over their chests. Max dropped his hands to his sides already exhausted. "Fuck. Are you always like this when you're together?"

"You wanna be around when it's the four of us," Riley snorted before adding reverently, "It's beautiful."

"Four Moore brothers," Max retorted, pulling his shades off. "Christ, your poor mother. I'm amazed she hasn't been committed."

"There's time yet," Tate said, nonchalantly patting Max on the shoulder. "So, come on, what's the deal?"

Max shook his head stubbornly. He ordered his coffee and his sandwich and, once he'd paid, he sat down with his tray at his usual spot, allowing himself a quiet moment to think about Grace and what she was doing in DC. She'd been gone a couple of days and, even with a few texts sent between them and Max keeping himself busy working with his uncle and painting, her absence was still noticeable. He wasn't sure he liked it all that much.

Tate and Riley sat down across from him with their food, drinks, and questioning expressions, looking like the damned Gestapo. "So spill, dude, come on," Riley said, punching his straw into a carton of orange juice. "Since when do we not share?"

Max frowned. "Like, ever. We never share because you couldn't keep a secret if it promised you hourly blow jobs."

Tate barked a laugh around his bagel, garnering a hurt glance from Riley.

"That's not true," Riley grumbled toward his plate of waffles and pancakes.

"It *is* fucking true," Max replied.

"It's okay, Riley," Tate said nonchalantly. "It's obvious that Max and Grace are more than just running partners now." He sipped his coffee. "It's written all over him."

Max dropped back in his seat casually, mouth full of sandwich. "Yeah. Okay. I fucked her. So what?"

"How many times?" Riley asked quickly, leaning forward.

Max frowned. "What?"

"O'Hare."

"Twice, why?"

"Ha!" Riley boomed, shoving Tate's shoulder with his own. "Pay up."

Tate grumbled under his breath while he pulled out his wallet and handed Riley a twenty. Max stared at the two of them in disbelief. "How— What did? You made a fucking bet?" His eyes flew back to the sandwich counter, where he'd left them both for mere moments.

Riley laughed unashamedly. "Of course, man, don't you know me at all?"

Max's attention snapped to Tate. "And you let him?"

Tate shrugged and tucked back into his bagel. "He promised to buy me a muffin and I'm a sugar whore."

Max dragged a hand down his face. "You amaze me."

"Not the first time I've been told that," Riley commented before slurping his juice hard enough to make the carton crumple in his hand. "So you two, like, a couple now?"

Max shook his head. "No. Not at all."

"So friends with benefits?" Tate asked, his eyes still on his food.

Max nodded, staring at Tate's red T-shirt, which read "Genius, Billionaire, Playboy, Philanthropist" in large yellow lettering.

"No," Riley uttered, following Max's line of sight. "I don't get it, either."

"Thank God," Max replied.

"Yeah," Riley continued. "I mean, why the fuck would you like Marvel when DC's where it's at?" He lifted his gray T-shirt to show the black long-sleeved top underneath emblazoned with a Batman symbol.

"Don't start," Tate said evenly. "We had this conversation on the way here."

"Yeah, we did," Riley answered with a smug smile, adjusting his clothes. "A conversation *you* lost."

"Well," Tate said, patting his lips delicately with his napkin. "That depends on your definition, now, doesn't it?"

Max's eyes snapped from one man to the other as if seated in center court, Wimbledon. "Dare I ask?"

"Tate believes that, in a fight, Captain America would beat Superman, which, any true comic book fan will tell you, would not happen."

"Cap has the shield," Tate said indifferently.

"Superman's bulletproof; what the fuck would a shield do?"

"Who the fuck cares?" Max interrupted.

After a beat of silence, the two men looked over at him as though he'd dropped out of the sky naked.

"Why do we even speak to him?" Riley asked, turning to his brother.

Tate sighed as though genuinely baffled. "I ask myself that every time I come here."

Max couldn't fight the smile that pulled at his mouth. "You two are batshit."

Riley pointed at him. "To be continued," he stated before he stood and made his way across the coffee shop toward the bathroom.

Tate waited until the door of the bathroom swung shut. "So, come on." He leaned his forearms on the table between them. "Before Boy Wonder comes back. What's really going on? You okay?"

Max shrugged. "Yeah, I'm okay. Good, actually." He smirked. "I mean who wouldn't be, having a hot woman to play with, huh?"

Tate didn't laugh along. "And she's of the same mind? She seemed pretty fond of you when I saw you with her."

"She understands," Max countered, swallowing a lump of something that felt like a lie.

"Is this a good idea?" Tate asked, seemingly sensing Max's discomfort. "You two."

"You've changed your tune." Max shook his head. "Besides, there is no us two. It's just sex."

Tate nodded, chewing the inside of his mouth. "I know the docs say that having a relationship in the first year of rehabilitation is a bad idea, but—"

"Jesus." Max exhaled an incredulous sound. "Wasn't that what I said to you? There is no relationship. We're just fuckin'. Seriously, man, I'm not getting involved with her or anyone. I don't want that." He licked his lips and glanced down at his half-eaten sandwich, his appetite dissolving slowly. "I don't ever want that. I can't."

Tate cleared his throat and sat back. He pressed his mouth into a tight line. "Okay."

Max narrowed his eyes. "Okay?"

"Yeah," Tate answered, lifting one shoulder. "If that's how it is, then that's how it is."

Max cocked his head to one side. "Why do I feel like you're fucking with me?"

"I'm not, Max. I wouldn't do that." Tate crossed his arms over his chest. "As your sponsor and as your friend, I have to make sure you're all right and that the choices you make are beneficial to your recovery." He shrugged. "If you tell me you're okay with this, that this is what you want, then fine. I'll support you."

Max dipped his chin in acquiescence, shaking off the suspicious feeling prickling his skin while allowing Tate's words of support to settle into him. He was surprised to realize that they made him feel better, more relaxed, as though Tate's blessing was somehow important to what was going on between him and Grace.

Grace.

Max sipped his coffee, thinking about how their dynamic had changed over the last couple of weeks. Damn, she was something else: passionate, demanding, and altogether hot as hell. The latter wasn't news, but combined with her newfound inner sex goddess, Grace was truly incredible. She liked everything he'd done to her and, despite her shy smile and fidgeting hands, she wasn't afraid to ask for what she wanted. Like the other day when she'd begged him to come all over her, just like he had in his room at the boardinghouse.

Max had worried that, despite the opposite intent, Grace would think his coming on her was degrading or demeaning or even, he shuddered at the thought, insulting. But when, lying on his bed, he'd seen the fire in her eyes and heard the husky plea leave her lips, he knew she liked it. She'd liked it even better the second time. They'd just gotten back from a run when Grace was sweating and breathless while stretching out on her carpet. Max had approached her, hard-on obvious in his running shorts, rubbing himself while he watched her.

Neither of them had spoken when she realized what he was doing. She hadn't even looked surprised, more pleased than outraged. It hadn't taken long for Grace's hand to travel between her legs and Max had watched as she made herself come, begging for him to do the same all over her.

Max had been more than happy to oblige, growling as his orgasm snapped up his spine, thrusting his hips out and pulsing his pleasure across Grace's body, the white of his come stretched across her dark caramel skin causing a deep, dark ball of possessiveness to curl in his chest.

Max hadn't given himself time to truly ponder—for reasons that were blatantly obvious—but it had been oddly intimate standing over her, touching himself while Grace did the same, the room silent but for their grunts and curses.

"How's the painting going?" Tate asked, his wry voice pulling Max back to his seat in the coffee shop.

Max cleared his throat and shifted in his chair. "Good. I'm painting nearly every day. When I get the time."

His paintings, just recently, had become a cacophony of vibrant colors and indiscernible patterns. He'd started to favor warmer colors, hotter colors, the usual blacks and grays of his initial artwork slowly fading into the background to make way for the golds, reds, and greens that tore across his canvases. The damn things seemed to create themselves with little help from the man holding the paintbrush. It seemed getting laid was all the creative motivation Max had needed. He smiled to himself. Hell. The curve of Grace's neck as she called out to God when they fucked, the smooth skin of her inner thighs, and the taste of her between them were completely inspiring. He checked his watch, wondering again what time tomorrow she'd be coming back from her trip to DC and whether she'd be up for round three.

"That's good, Max," Tate commented, his eyes on Max's watch when Max looked up. "You late for something?" He smirked when Max flipped him the bird.

"Okay," Riley said and thumped back down into his seat. "What awesome sexy-time details did I miss?" He shoved a huge forkful of waffle into his mouth.

"None," Max said, leaning forward. "Anyway, forget that, I need to talk to you about Carter's bachelor party." He lifted his eyebrows. "Any ideas?"

The smile that spread across Riley's face was huge. "Dude," he mumbled around his food. "Do you even need to ask? I have links on my phone." He began riffling in his jeans pocket.

Max snickered into his coffee cup, not feeling guilty at all for using Riley's short attention span to his advantage. He knew he'd successfully dodged a barrage of questions he had neither the forbearance nor inclination to answer, while avoiding Tate's knowing stare needling him across the table.

•   •   •

"Grace?"

Grace opened her eyes slowly, scared to death that the room would tilt horrifically should she do it too quickly. She immediately grimaced. The pounding in her head, along with the nausea that gripped her entire body, made her pull the duvet closer, cocooning herself in her sweats, hoodie, and socks. That was the second time she'd woken thinking that she'd heard Max's voice. Hallucinations no doubt brought on by the hundred-degree temperatures that had spiked in the early hours. She couldn't understand it; she was so cold her teeth chattered.

"Grace?"

The voice sounded louder now, closer. She hummed into her pillow, shivering and mumbling, wishing that Max really *was* there so she could snuggle into him, get warm next to him, maybe grope him a little.

"Grace, are you in here, we're supposed to be on our run— Jesus Christ! What the hell?"

Yeah, that sounded like him, all curse words and exclamations. Wait. A run? Some part of her understood what she was hearing, knew what the words meant, but her brain was so very tired. She couldn't find it in herself to respond. Instead, she smiled to herself, the image of Max running flashing behind her eyes.

There was a sound of a window being opened and gust of fresh air hit her face, making Grace squirm and bury her head farther under the covers. "It's like a fucking sauna in here! And shit—is that puke I smell?"

Yeah, it probably was. Grace could vaguely remember vomiting a few times on herself, before she'd managed to muster the energy to change out her bedsheets, but not enough to crawl into the shower. Her legs had been far too weak. She couldn't recall, however, how long ago that had been. It could have been days. She almost cared that Max, hallucination or not, was near her when she was full of sick bits, but she couldn't gather enough energy to tell him to go away.

"Are you awake?" The duvet was pulled gently from her grasp, causing another violent shiver to gallop across her. She gasped when something large and freezing cold touched her forehead. "Shit, Grace, you're burning up."

Maybe he was real. "Max?" The cover disappeared altogether. Grace tried to protest, tried to reach for it, but her body just wouldn't move. "Don't," she mumbled, opening her eyes into small slits, seeing a blur of dark hair and darker eyes. "Cold."

"You're not cold," the dark eyes told her. "You have a fever. Come on."

She cried out when hands grabbed at her and hauled her into strong arms. "I know. I'm sorry," he said soothingly. She hurt everywhere he touched. God, she wanted her momma.

"Shhh," he whispered against her cheek. "I've got you." His hand was icy on her face. "Don't cry."

"It hurts," she croaked against the nausea, slumping against him.

"I know," he murmured. "I'm going to try and cool you down, okay?"

"Max?"

"Yeah."

"I think I was sick."

He chuckled. "Yeah, I think you were."

"Don't smell me."

"Too late."

"Oh God."

"Don't worry about it. We're going to take a shower, all right?" A shower sounded cold. She shook her head. "Please, don't."

"It'll feel colder than it is because you're so hot. Jesus, Grace, you're shaking, why the hell didn't you call?"

She didn't know. The last thing she remembered was getting home last night from DC feeling more tired than usual, with a splitting headache, and crawling into bed. Then her dinner had made a reappearance and everything went tits up.

"I'm gonna sit you down. Hold on to me."

Grace's backside hit something cool and she tilted sideways, caught by Max's hand on her shoulder. She didn't have the strength to hold on to him. Her fingers just wouldn't work.

"Hey."

"Hey," she muttered back. "It hurts, Max. Can you—"

"Can you do me a favor?"

A favor! Was he nuts? She could barely sit up. She opened her eyes to see Max crouching in front of her, his handsome face serious. They were in the bathroom. She was sitting on the toilet seat. He had a cell phone to his ear. What the hell was going on?

"I'm at Grace's. I found her in bed. She's running a really high fever . . . no, she's not really with it." His hands found her face again. "She can't hold herself up— No, she's not. Yeah, she's definitely puked. I was going to put her in the shower, try and cool her down . . . okay. I don't have the number. Can you call him? Thanks."

"I'm sorry," she whispered as he slipped his cell back into the pocket of his shorts, the urge to cry again scratching her throat.

"For being ill?" he asked, standing up in front of her. "Don't be dumb. Lift your arms for me."

She did as he asked without question and hissed when the frigid air of the bathroom hit her skin. "Please, Max." She shivered. "I need my sweater."

"After you've showered with me. Lift up so I can pull off your sweats." She wobbled when she stood and he held her upright. "You should be ecstatic," he added from her feet. "You told me you wanted me to have you in the shower."

She closed her eyes and groaned as her stomach rolled and the room swam. "Max, you're very pretty, but I don't think we can have sex right now."

His laugh was beautiful but it hurt her ears and made her head pulse. She closed her eyes.

"Don't worry, Gracie, I just want to help make you feel better."

His nickname for her made her smile. He lifted her again, his body like ice against hers, and moved them both into the shower. She whimpered and clutched on to him as he turned the water on and the spray caught her foot like a rush of Arctic Ocean. She cried out, the sensation like a fierce slap against her skin.

"Max, please," she begged into his shoulder, trying her best to climb up him and away from the water.

"Hang on. It'll only be for a minute. I'll do it quickly. You need to cool down, sweetheart. You're far too hot." His lips pressed against her temple. "Hold me."

She cried out again when he lifted the showerhead and moved it hastily over her body, keeping it for long moments on the back of her neck and her scalp. It hurt. It hurt and made her bones vibrate, but she knew somewhere in the back of her heat-addled mind that it was for her own good. She sniffled and whimpered into Max's neck, hearing him turn off the water and step out of the shower. She was still in his arms and, when she opened her eyes, she could see goose bumps running across his shoulder.

"Ar-are you c-cold?" she stammered against her chattering teeth.

"I'm fine. Don't worry about me."

She couldn't help it, though. She cared for him, a whole lot, so worrying was part of the deal.

"Is that so?"

She nuzzled his neck, pretending she had not just said that aloud. Shit. A towel was swiftly wrapped around her and he placed her carefully on the circular love seat she had in her bedroom next to the large window he'd opened. She shook.

"Stay here while I change your bed, okay?"

"Sheets in th-the clos-set."

"I know," he whispered, his lips near her cheek.

She wished he'd kiss her. She wished he'd just stay and hold her. She wished she could appreciate seeing him wet from the shower. Wait. Was he naked? She tried to open her eyes, but they wouldn't cooperate. Instead, she snuggled against the cushions of the love seat and pulled the towel closer, trying to keep warm.

. . .

Max rolled over and was greeted with a fist smacking hard into his cheek. "Ow. Jeez!" He cursed and grumbled, grimacing as he clutched his face. "Shit, Grace."

From her side of her bed, Grace blinked up at him in surprise, her eyes tired and her hair a fuzzy disaster.

"I just slept here to make sure you were all right," he explained. "No need to beat me up."

She blinked at him again, seemingly lost and trying to piece together the last thirty-six hours. Max watched her carefully as he sat up against the wrought-iron headboard. At least she'd regained a little more color than she had had the day before. If it hadn't been for all the shivering and shaking and grumbling nonsense, Max would have thought she was dead when he found her. Damn woman had given him a heart attack.

Grace rubbed a hand down her face and shifted heavily so she, too, was sitting up. "Oh. Oh dear. I feel like crap."

"You look it," Max commented honestly.

Grace snorted. "Thanks."

He shrugged. "Just keeping it real. If it's any consolation you look a damn sight better than you did."

Grace sighed, grimacing with each movement. "Was I run over by a truck?" She ran her hands through her hair but froze midway through. "Oh God, I was sick. I was sick a lot." Her face was instantly mortified. "Max, that's twice you've cleaned me up while I was spewing."

"Tell me about it," Max replied earnestly. "It's a good thing one of us has a strong stomach."

She looked like she was going to cry. Max couldn't have handled that again. Once was bad enough. It had damn near broke his heart when, in her fever-riddled haze, she'd asked for her mother.

"I'm so sorry."

"Oh, stop," Max said with a breath of amusement. "It's fine." He took a deep breath. "Although, I have to admit, I was severely disappointed that you weren't wearing that red underwear again when I stripped you."

Grace's eyes widened. "Stripped me?"

"Mmhm," Max hummed, stretching; he caught her stare on his bare chest. "For the shower."

"Shower?"

Max chuckled and nodded. "Together." He winked. "Shame you were too ill to remember."

"Amen," Grace sighed, looking decidedly disappointed.

"Well, there's always next time." Max grinned. "Do you still feel sick?"

At his words, a loud gurgle emitted from Grace's stomach.

He cocked an eyebrow. "Hungry?"

Grace looked around herself. "Water?"

Max gestured toward the side table next to her, where there sat a large glass of water, a bottle of Gatorade, and a couple of white tablets. "It's just Tylenol. The doctor wanted to give you a shot of something but I didn't know if you were allergic or whether it would fuck with your meds, and I didn't much fancy a trip to the ER, so we just gave you some ibuprofen and Tylenol to bring your temperature down."

Grace finished the whole glass frowning. "Doctor?"

Max smiled. Yeah, she'd been totally out of it. "I called Aunt Fern, who called the doctor. Just a forty-eight-hour thing. He said you'll be fine. Thank God." He yawned. "I don't think I could handle sleeping here again with all of your damn twitching and mumbling."

It'd been like sleeping inside a damn washing machine and Max was genuinely surprised he didn't have more bruises. Initially, he'd grabbed a couple of blankets and bunkered down on the love seat, giving Grace the space to flail and turn in her bed. But, after a while, she'd started to cry out in her sleep, muttering nonsense that kept him awake for more than an hour. Tired and cranky, he'd scrambled into bed with her just after midnight and soothed her until her fever broke. As she had been after her panic attack in the bar, she was calm only when he was next to her, touching her. A fact that made something feel warm deep in his belly.

Grace looked at him, aghast. "What the hell was I say— Are you joking?"

He shook his head. "It was gibberish, mainly. Then it was about how awesome you think I am, how you can't live without me—" He laughed when Grace swatted weakly at him. It was almost the truth, though he'd never tell her. She'd slurred a few times as she snuggled into him about how much he meant to her, and how pretty he was. The former made parts of Max twitch in discomfort but the latter made him chuckle and shush her until she was snoring softly. Then the next bout of fidgeting and fighting with the covers would start.

Grace smiled, appeased, the worry fading from her eyes before she frowned. "Wait. What day is it? I have to work."

"Monday. I've been here since Sunday morning, when you didn't show for our run. And don't worry, I called Holly."

She exhaled, relieved. "Thank you. Shouldn't you be at work?"

Max shook his head. "Uncle Vince said I could play hooky, to make sure you were still breathing and shit. Besides, he owes me."

"He does?"

Max took a deep breath and licked his lips. "Josh and I with a few of the other guys are helping him on a job in Philly. A friend of his got behind schedule on a build and . . . we'll be staying there to get it done faster. It should take about a week, maybe ten days."

Grace blinked, her teeth worrying her bottom lip a little. "Oh."

Max wasn't sure why he'd felt guilty when his uncle had asked for his help and he'd said yes and why now, when he told Grace, he felt it again. "Yeah, we go on Thursday morning bright and early."

He tried to smile. "Hey, just think of all the peace and quiet you'll get while I'm away."

Grace breathed a small laugh but it fell flat between them, settling with a heavy silence that covered them both like a blanket. Max fidgeted at her side, the need to say something fighting with the urge he had to hug her. Her next question relieved him of doing either.

"How did you get in here?"

Shit. Max had been hoping that somehow that question would have passed her by. "Your hide-a-key."

Grace frowned. "But only my brother and Ruby know about that."

Max shifted nervously. "Yeah, about that, look, don't be mad at her, okay?"

"At who? Ruby?"

He nodded. "I don't want you to freak out, but I got worried when you didn't show or answer your phone and I didn't know if you were back from DC, because you hadn't called, so I came over. I didn't know if something had happened, because it looked like you were home, but you didn't come to the door. So I phoned Ruby and she told me where it was so I could get in and check on you." He paused and swallowed. "Sorry."

Grace smirked. "You're cute when you ramble."

"Am not."

"Are so." She waved a hand, stopping him from arguing further. "Why would I have freaked out?"

Max shrugged. "Strange man in your house without permission. I mean, I didn't want to assume you'd be okay with me doing that but I was—"

"Worried?"

Max narrowed his eyes at her smile and huffed. "Yeah. But I wish I hadn't bothered. I don't think I'll ever get the whiff of vomit off me."

Grace giggled and snorted incredulously as she said, "Strange man."

Max shook his head. She was definitely feeling better. "Whatever. I'm going to make some coffee." He threw his legs off the bed and thumped to the floor.

"Max?"

He stopped at the doorway and turned.

"Thank you for helping me. Really."

Max dipped his chin, her sincerity and wide, innocent eyes yanking the grumpiness from him and replacing it with something warmer, something that would allow Grace to get away with just about anything. It was so good to see her.

"You're welcome." He exhaled and threw a thumb over his shoulder. "You want something?"

"Penicillin," Grace muttered.

"What?"

"I'm allergic to penicillin. You know? Just in case this happens again."

Max snorted. "Christ. I hope not. But thanks. That's good to know."

"Any time, Rambler."

"Shut up." Max turned and headed out of the room. "Vomit Face."

24

By Wednesday, Grace was feeling her normal self again. Max had been an angel, all but bending over backward to make sure she had everything she wanted or needed to make her better. He'd stayed until she'd fallen asleep on Monday night after making her toast and tea for lunch, leaving her to snooze while he watched TV and even running her a bath when Grace complained that she could no longer cope with her own gross, sweaty smell. The only negative was that Max had ignored her unsubtle requests for him to join her in the lavender bubbles. He'd grumbled about her being the death of him and left her to soak.

She'd woken Tuesday morning to a handwritten note on the pillow next to her:

> *Hope you slept. I left a muffin and a latte on the kitchen counter. I'm helping my uncle but I'll call over later and see how you are. Max.*

Grace tried to curtail the butterflies that swarmed as she read his note over and over, trying like hell to not see the caring words as anything more than a friend helping another friend, but it was futile. She was falling faster and harder than she'd ever dared to hope for again and she had no way of stopping it.

"Penny for them," Holly asked, bumping her hip against Grace's as Grace's towel did another circuit of the bar.

Grace startled, knocking a half-filled glass of Heineken and catching it before it toppled completely, earning a smirk from Earl, a huff from Caleb, and a knowing giggle from Holly. Grace had no idea how long she'd been standing there, drifting into space with only her thoughts of Max to keep her company. She felt her cheeks heat and scurried away to serve a couple of regulars.

"Hey, Grace!" Ruby's voice echoed from the entrance as she all but skipped through it. She was still in her coveralls, covered in grease, having obviously come straight from work, a small pink bow bouncing in her hair. Grace smiled. She still had no idea how such a girly girl as Ruby could love getting so messy while working on the cars she did. It was a dichotomy to which Grace had warmed quickly.

"So, with Josh being away, you know what that means, right?" Ruby literally vibrated where she stood. "Girls' night!"

Caleb turned to them both from his usual seat at the bar. "Away?"

"Yeah," Ruby answered. "They're helping Dad's friend in Philly. He's taking a team of them." She turned back to Grace. "Well?"

Grace laughed, popping the cap and placing a bottle of Diet Pepsi in front of her. "Sounds . . . interesting."

Ruby rolled her eyes. "Oh, come on. You can't mope for the next week while Max is gone."

Grace's shoulders snapped back when Holly and Ruby shared a look. Caleb cleared his throat and eyed her over the lip of his glass as he drained it. "I wouldn't—why would I? Don't be silly."

She blatantly ignored the snickering coming from the others sitting around the bar, who apparently knew that she would, indeed, be wallowing and missing Max like crazy while he was gone. Jesus, she was so transparent and this town was too damn small. "Fine," she said, blinking slowly. "I'm in."

Ruby grinned. "Awesome. I'll call the girls and arrange something for this weekend. Storms are forecast next week so we need to plan now."

"Storms?"

Ruby waved her off. "Just a little thunder and lightning. We usually get a good few days of them. Clears the air real good." She sipped the rest of her drink, threw a bill on the bar, and started walking backward toward where she'd appeared. "Now excuse me while I go and abuse my husband in all the ways he loves before he leaves tomorrow."

Grace laughed, shaking her head and wondering whether she'd get the chance to abuse Max in all the ways *he* loved before he left. With that thought, however, instead of excitement, she was suddenly struck with an intense feeling of melancholy. This work trip with Vince had brought home the very real prospect that Max wasn't going to be around Preston County forever.

Grace knew he had a life in New York, friends who were close enough to warrant being called family. His best friend was getting married soon and he was going to be best man. He had a life waiting for him and Grace had to wonder whether she'd factor into any of it when he decided to return. Of course, in terms of romance, she knew that it was an impossibility; Max had made that clear. But could they remain friends or would Max simply take off and leave without a second glance?

"Grace, honey."

Swallowing down her uneasiness for another day, Grace looked over to Holly, who was holding the draft pump at a ninety-degree angle, getting nothing but gurgling foam. "Can you go down and change the keg out?"

Grace smiled wanly. "Sure."

She dropped her towel to the bar and headed toward the stone steps, located at the back of the building She went down to the cellar, flicking on lights as she went. The place had always given her the heebie-jeebies—God alone knew what creepy-crawlies hung out in the nooks and crannies of the place—but she was slowly getting used to it. As long as she could hear the people in the bar above, she didn't start to panic.

After fighting with a box of Coke syrup, she finally located the empty barrel and rolled another one into its place, reattaching the pipe and calling out an "Okay" for Holly to start pumping.

"Loud little thing, aren't you?"

Grace squeaked in surprise, whirling around, hand clutched to her chest to find Max smirking in that devastatingly handsome way of his, leaning nonchalantly against one of the cellar's support columns. He was filthy. His arms were caked in dirt and she could see smudges on his face where he'd wiped at the sweat he'd no doubt worked up. It had been a scorcher of a day. His blue jeans were blackened, as was his gray T-shirt, which stretched gorgeously across his chest. She imagined he smelled incredible, all musky and man. He was the sexiest thing she'd ever seen.

"What are you doing down here?" she asked, her voice shaking with the adrenaline still coursing through her. She wasn't scared, of course, but the way Max was staring at her made her body tighten in ways that were altogether delicious.

His stare strayed back up to the steps to the basement door, which was still open a crack. He smirked and dropped his chin, his stare predatory. "Imagine my delight when Holly said you were down here. All."

He took a step toward her. "By."

Another. "Yourself."

Grace's back hit cold stone. Her chest heaved. "And why would that delight you?"

He paused, his gaze snapping from her denim skirt to her face. "Because I vividly remember you saying, while you were riding me, that you'd thought about me fucking you here."

Grace remembered, too. God, she remembered everything from that day. The first time he slipped inside her and whispered her name as though it were a prayer. The feel of his hands so tight on her hips, the sound of his skin slapping against hers, and the twitch of his orgasm inside of her.

Her recollecting that perfect day must have appeared like hesitancy, and the fire and want in Max's dark eyes died a little.

"I'm sorry," he blurted. "I'm an idiot." His hand found his hair quickly. "I just thought that we could, because you said— But if you don't—"

"Max?" Grace interrupted, moving her hands to the edge of her denim skirt, heat lurching across her skin.

He watched her movements like a hawk, swallowing when she lifted it, showing him her underwear. "Oh shit. Yeah?"

"Shut up and fuck me."

He was on her in moments, yanking her panties down, dropping to his knees, and burying his face between her legs. Grace cried out before slamming her forearm against her mouth. His tongue was perfect, so damned perfect, and when he . . . oh, God, did that thing against her clit, she about fell apart in his hands. He was voracious and, once again, Grace fantasized about what his mouth against hers would be like. She wanted to taste his tongue so badly. Would he be as hungry? What would his lips feel like as he came? Would he—she called out—kiss her . . . just. Like. That?

"I want you," she managed, gasping, vaguely aware that voices from the bar were drifting down to them through the open door.

Max eyes lit further. He pulled his mouth from her. "Yes. How? Tell me how."

His deep voice and the way it curled around her with lust and desire sparked something in Grace that she'd thought long lost. Her back straightened and her chin lifted as confidence and sexiness began to fill her so quickly, she thought she might burst.

This man. This beautiful man on his knees before her *wanted* her. *Really* wanted her. He wanted to please her, to make her feel good. And at that moment it didn't matter to Grace how long that might be for. No, he wouldn't be in West Virginia forever and that hurt and scared her more than she could possibly allow it to, but at that very moment, from the look on his face, wet with her need for him, she knew he would have done anything she'd asked.

Grace turned, placing her palms against the wall, and arched, pushing her ass toward him. "Like this."

"Fucking Christ," he muttered, not moving but for his hands, which ghosted so carefully over her skin, cupping her hips, and trailing his thumbs between her cheeks. He breathed deeply and grunted when his teeth scraped across her ass. "You're not playing fair," he muttered.

"I don't want to play," Grace answered. "I just want to feel you."

She felt his lips against her butt before he stood abruptly. The sound of his heavy belt clanging as he undid it made goose bumps pop up along Grace's arms. He pressed against her, his cock hard against her thigh.

"Can you keep quiet?" he grunted before he ripped open the condom wrapper with his teeth.

"No," she gasped honestly.

He laughed darkly. "Good, because I want them all to hear what I do to you."

Grace's entire body shivered.

"Shhh, it's all right," he whispered next to her ear, his nose trailing up the lobe while his tongue darted out to lick her neck. "I've got you." He pressed his large hands to the small of her back and, for a brief moment, his voice lost its husk, becoming careful, concerned. "You okay?"

Grace's eyes rolled at that. "Yes. Please," she whimpered, pushing back. "I need you."

The tip of his cock brushed against her. "How do you need me?"

"Hard." The word slipped from her mouth before Grace even had the urge to say it, but it was the God's honest truth. She wanted him to fuck her, and fuck her hard. She wanted to feel him inside her for days so that she wouldn't feel so damned hollow when he left in the morning.

"That's my girl." He was inside her in one swift movement, dragging a groan from them both and lifting Grace almost to her tiptoes. He was perfect, filling her almost to the point of discomfort until he pulled his hips back and pushed in again. She mewed with each thrust and gasped his name as he panted in her ear. He was careful not to crowd her, not to hold her against the wall so that she'd panic, and she adored him all the more for it.

"Will you think about this?" he asked, slamming into her again, his hands lusciously tight on her hips. "While I'm away. Will you think about my cock in you?"

Grace loved the beautiful filth that tumbled from his mouth. She dropped her head back to his shoulder. "Yes."

"Will you miss it?"

I'll miss you.

"So much."

He moaned and moved his hands from her hips to her breasts, fighting with her vest top to get under her bra. He squeezed, his fingers pinching her skin. "You feel so good on my cock." His forehead met her shoulder, as though he was watching himself move in her. "Look at you taking me. You're so beautiful, Gracie. You fuck so good."

He mumbled and murmured words so dirty and unintentionally tender that Grace's eyes began to sting with the threat of tears. "Oh."

"Yeah?" Max asked, taking her desperate sound as a reason to tilt his hips and find that place inside of her that he knew would have her coming in moments.

"More," she begged, vaguely aware that her voice was getting louder. "Please, Max, more."

With a loud growl, Max slammed into her again and again, cursing and grunting and sweating against her. His fingers found her clit to rub and tease and get her there faster until, with a shout, he came, holding her so tightly to his chest that, when Grace's orgasm smashed into her not two seconds later and her legs weakened with its force, she didn't hit the floor. He held her to him, his breaths heavy and loud in her ear, as she squeezed him inside her, knowing that he would pull out quickly but wanting, no, *needing* him to stay inside her longer.

He made sure she was capable of holding herself up when he slowly pulled his body from hers. She took a second to rest her forehead against the wall and laughed, watching him over her shoulder. She'd never felt more energized despite the fatigue that clutched her muscles. Max smiled back, discarding the condom with a tissue he pulled from his pocket in a nearby trash can, and zipped himself up. He drifted closer to her, his palm smoothing across her ass at the same time a sated and sensual growl rumbled in his chest.

"Look at you," he murmured. "So sexy. I love that I'm the only one who gets to see you like this."

Grace couldn't be sure if the hint of covetousness in his voice was real or of her own imagination. His dark gaze settled on hers before he leaned forward and placed a gentle kiss at the corner of her mouth. It was the closest he'd ever been to kissing her properly and Grace's breath caught.

"You okay?" he asked, pulling back and helping her turn around while she fixed her skirt.

She smiled and nodded, watching as he bent down and picked her panties up from the floor. He held them up, looking at them with a hint of dark playfulness.

"What?"

"I'm a little torn," he confessed. "I want nothing more than to put these in my pocket and take them with me, so I can touch them while I'm away from you." Grace gaped. "But the idea of you being pantyless while you're working with Deputy AssCrack sitting at the bar makes me want to rip his eyeballs out of their sockets."

He handed them over with a small smile edged with embarrassment. Whether it was because of what he'd just admitted wasn't clear, but Grace couldn't have cared less. His words made her feel nothing but blissful and altogether shameless. Take her panties *with him*? Christ, the man knew exactly what to say to make her insanely hot.

It was such a strange paradox. Rick had, during their marriage, been a controlling, possessive asshole who continually told Grace that she *belonged* to him, that she was his to treat as he wanted. It had been awful, degrading, and had caused Grace to feel worthless. But when Max allowed his possessiveness to slip out, as he had each time they'd been intimate, it created a smolder within Grace, a deep heat that settled in her bones and made her want to take him to bed and help him see that he could love again if he just let her in.

She felt anything but worthless when Max looked at her.

She pulled on her underwear and fixed her clothes as best as she could. Max snickered behind his hand.

"Stop it," she chastised with a smirk, knowing that she would still look thoroughly humped no matter what she did. Not that she cared. If the bar patrons hadn't heard them, they'd been gone long enough for them all to figure it out. She sighed and crossed her arms over her chest, feeling the cold outside of Max's embrace. "What time do you leave in the morning?"

"Six." Max pushed his hands into his pockets and rocked on his heels. "I'm gonna head back to the boardinghouse, get some food, and call it a night."

Grace nodded. "Okay." She watched him carefully as he opened his mouth and then closed it again.

"You'll be okay getting home on your own tonight?"

He usually took her home when she worked late at the bar. She smiled and nodded. "Can I . . . while you're gone—can I text you?"

The side of Max's mouth lifted. "Sure. Call if you want."

"Okay."

"Okay," he echoed. "I . . ." He paused, uncharacteristically fidgety. He wiped a palm across his forehead and an uncertain laugh burst from him. "Shit, okay, I'm outta here." He half-turned away from her. "Are you sure it was all right that I, that we— You're fine?"

His rambling never ceased to endear him further to Grace. "It was very fine."

Max licked his lips. "Damn straight, girl." He grinned and turned fully. "Speak to you soon," he called as he took the cellar steps two at a time, only to be greeted by rapturous applause, cheers, and catcalls when he pushed his way through the door and back into the bar.

·   ·   ·

Knock, knock.

Who's there?

Adore.

Adore who?

Adore is between us. Open up!

Grace. Seriously.

Knock, knock.

Really?

Come on. Knock, knock.

Who's there!?

Harry.

Harry who?

Harry up, it's cold out here!

That's it, I'm blocking you.

You'd never.

You're probably right.

Grace grinned down at her phone before sliding it into the front pocket of her apron. She'd been abusing Max with her dad's old knock-knock jokes for two days and he was still humoring her, God bless him. It was Saturday and, after her run, Grace had locked herself in her darkroom to work on her gallery collection, the deadline for which was looming quietly.

She hummed and bobbed her head slowly to Marvin Gaye's *Trouble Man*, her favorite album for when she was developing photographs. She picked up one particular shot with her tweezers and let the developing solution run off it. It was a favorite of hers, taken of Max, unaware that she'd taken the picture. It was July Fourth while they were hanging by the lake. He was smiling, his eyes creasing in that adorable way of his, his laughter almost audible from the print. There was no hint of the pain or struggle that Max had endured. He looked truly peaceful, truly beautiful.

Grace fastened it to the line that hung from one corner of her darkroom to the other with a small clip and stood back, observing the shots she was to use in her collection as well as those she'd decided to hide and keep for herself. The latter were mostly of Max. That man had a face made for film.

Her phone buzzed in her pocket. Max.

Knock, knock!

Who's there?

Ivana.

Ivana who?

Ivana hump your brains out!

Grace snorted.

I wish you could. But you're not here. For now, I guess, I'll have to pleasure myself.

The three small gray dots on her cell screen flickered and then disappeared, as though he was typing then deleting repeatedly, before his reply finally came through: *Damn. Are you really?*

She laughed while typing: No. No time, although I may do that later. I have to get ready for my girls' night. Bet you wish you'd taken my panties now, don't you?

• • • •

"Wow, Max, you look like you've seen a ghost. Everything all right?"

Max looked up from his cell phone to Josh, who was sitting

across the table of the burger and grill place the team had chosen to eat. There were twelve of them at a long table in the center of the place, all of them talking and ravenous from the day's labor. Max ached in places he'd forgotten about since his gym sessions in rehab. It was no wonder he hurt, considering all the lifting and lugging he'd done over the past few days.

"What's up?" Josh asked, looking at the phone in Max's hand.

Max shoved his cell into the pocket of his jeans, which were a little snug thanks to Grace's message. Shit. He'd created a monster. "Just a text from Grace."

Josh raised an eyebrow. "Yeah, I can tell what kind of text, too. Ruby is a nightmare for that when I'm away and can't do anything about it."

Max grimaced. "Dude, that's my cousin."

"And my daughter," Vince called from three places down above the noise.

Josh sat forward, ignoring his father-in-law. "So, you and Grace, huh?"

"What about me and Grace?"

Josh shrugged nonchalantly, avoiding Max's pointed stare, smiling down at his pot of ranch dressing. "I just heard you guys had fun at Whiskey's the other night."

"Everyone heard," Rob added from next to Max, nudging him playfully. The other guys nearest to them smirked. They'd obviously heard about Max and Grace's cellar activities, too.

Max grinned despite himself. He knew the banter would come eventually and, truthfully, he didn't mind. It wasn't like he was embarrassed. *Hell* no.

Seeing the deputy's eyes fire up when he emerged from the cellar with the smell of Grace all over him?

That shit was golden. He'd all but sauntered past the prick with a smirk front and center. Besides, he knew Grace hadn't been too uncomfortable that they'd been heard. She'd known it was a possibility and, Christ, she'd practically begged him for it. He exhaled and picked up his fork, recollecting that shit-hot look she'd given him over her shoulder. It was filled with a dare, a want, and all the things that made Max want to do dastardly things to her wherever and whenever they could. Woman was dangerous without even trying.

He paused, and played with the food on his plate. He knew deep down he should have felt unsettled, but he couldn't find it in himself—beneath the unfamiliar sensation of contentment that had snuck in since Grace arrived on the scene—to care. Grace was fun to fuck. She was gorgeous, and witty, and he liked being around her. He liked *her*. He liked what they were doing and for the first time in a while, he liked what it felt like. Their arrangement worked and he was enjoying himself. Plus, he was eight months clean and sober. With no worries, no strings, and with the heavy weight of his addiction gradually becoming lighter and easier to bear as each day passed, life felt pretty damn awesome.

"You're a lucky son of a bitch," Rob muttered under his breath. "She's smoking hot."

"Aren't you married?" another guy, whose name Max couldn't recall, and who had cornrows and sparkling white teeth, asked from Rob's other side.

"Please," Rob countered with a shrug. "Just 'cause I'm eatin', don't mean I can't look at the menu."

Max picked up his cheeseburger and took a mammoth bite, not even the least bit guilty for enjoying the sliver of smugness that wrapped around his chest.

"So are you guys, like, exclusive?" Josh asked, sipping from his beer bottle.

Max shook his head. "We're not a couple or anything, it's casual, but we don't sleep with anyone else."

"Damn. There goes my shot," Josh's friend Aiden drawled, snapping his fingers. He looked at Max with attentive gray eyes, his blond eyebrows furrowing playfully. "Wait. How long you stayin' in Preston County? When do you go back to New York?"

The table laughed again at Aiden's suggestion, but for some reason, Max struggled to join in. He smiled faintly at Josh as he shook his head good-naturedly at his friend, and picked up his drink, rubbing the heel of his hand against a sudden heat burning deep in the center of his chest. He eyed his burger distrustfully.

Damn indigestion.

· · · ·

A few hours later, after leaving the majority of the guys propping up a whiskey bar in the city, Max headed back to the small but comfortable hotel they had been put up in. It wasn't that watching other people get shitfaced while he stayed sober wasn't super-duper fun, but there was only so much Max could resist before the scent of bourbon developed into a siren's call.

He'd called Tate as he walked the four blocks, explaining where he was and what he'd been doing. It was a casual conversation—they shot the shit, he dodged questions about Grace, and they caught up—but Max could hear the underlying concern in Tate's voice that appeared whenever Max called unexpectedly. Months ago the sound of it would have had his molars grinding, but now he found himself smiling. It was a good feeling having people on his side.

Throwing himself down on his hotel bed and switching on the TV, Max glanced at his watch. It was a little before midnight. He tapped his cell screen against his knuckle, wondering whether Grace would still be up. She'd said something about a girls' night so it was entirely possible. With a shrug he started typing out a text.

Back at the hotel. How was your night?

He sent it, threw the phone down on the bed, and heaved himself up and to the bathroom to clean up before he went to bed. He heard his phone vibrate as he finished brushing his teeth. He wandered back into the room, pulling his Henley over his head and kicking his boots to the corner of the room. He picked up his phone and frowned at the text.

Kmoxk Knixk

"What the hell?" Max smirked.

Seems someone has been at the cocktails again.

Yupl

Be safe. Have fun.

I wush you ware here. O miss yo.

Max chuckled while trying to ignore the warm sensation whispering across his neck.

Put your drink down and go home. I'll call you tomorrow.

Home goin now. Yo mish me toooooooooo!!!!

Max snickered at the numerous heart-eye emojis at the end of her message and shook his head. He put his cell on charge, resisting the urge to text her back.

It didn't matter in any case; they both knew she was right.

25

As forecast, the storm rolled in at seven o'clock Friday evening of the following week.

It arrived with a ferocious roar and streaks of lightning followed by rain, the likes of which Grace had never seen. The humidity that had built over the past few days had been so brutal, like breathing water through a sieve, that Grace had given up even attempting to run while it hung around. Instead, to pass the time when she wasn't behind the bar, she cranked up the AC and worked on her photographs.

A flash of lightning illuminated Whiskey's, setting the lights to flickering. Grace jumped from her spot by the fridge and looked toward the window. It had been in full flow for a good hour with no sign of letting up. It was going to be all sorts of fun getting home tonight.

For a Friday, Whiskey's was all but empty except for Earl, Caleb, who'd just finished his shift, and a couple of regulars who spent so much time in Whiskey's, Grace wasn't sure they remembered where they lived anymore. Word had gotten around so quickly about the oncoming storm that even hot wings and liquor couldn't entice the masses. Folks had the right idea. The only reason Grace was working was that Holly was unwell, seemingly a victim of the dreaded sickness bug that had made Grace's life a misery more than a week ago.

Thunder shook the bar. Grace's eyes widened and Caleb chuckled. "Ah, don't you worry none. This is tame compared to our usual summer storms," he offered. "You'll be fine."

Grace wasn't so sure. She was just relieved that Max and the rest of the guys weren't heading back to Preston County until Sunday, when the storm was forecast to be at its weakest. Roads would be treacherous and she'd do nothing but spend her time worrying about him getting back safely otherwise. She poured herself a soda.

Lord. She couldn't wait to see him. It had seemed like the longest eight days of her life. They'd texted and even spoken on the phone a couple of times—even though Grace could sense Max's awkwardness when they did—but it wasn't the same.

An almighty crack of thunder that sounded as though it was directly above the bar snapped out the lights for a brief moment. A car alarm wailed somewhere outside as though crying out in surprise. Despite it nearing the end of July, the sky was black as rain barrelled down onto the ground below.

"Maybe I should close up?" Grace muttered, eyeing the wavering strip lights and glancing around at the faces sitting at the bar. Surprisingly, they all looked to be of the same opinion despite it being before 9 p.m. "We'd all be safer at home, right?"

Caleb slapped his hands on the bar, moving his bottle of Coke out of the way. "You're right. I'll head upstairs, tell Holly what we're doing, and drop each of you off in the cruiser. That thing could drive through just about anything."

Earl wheezed. "Cruiser, huh? Not been in the back of one of them since I was younger'n you."

Grace turned back to Caleb. "If you're sure."

He nodded and disappeared up the back steps to Holly's place. While he was gone, Grace cleaned up, thankful that the bar had been so quiet. She switched off all the electrics—save for the fridges—remembering her mother saying something about electrical sockets and storms not mixing, and stood with the other patrons at the door, waiting patiently for Caleb.

After locking the door and pushing the keys through the mailbox, Grace squealed and slid to the police cruiser, scrambling into the front seat before the rain could saturate every part of her. It was a losing battle. She pushed back hair that dripped down her nose, amazed that in mere moments the storm had left her looking like she'd been in the shower. "Ballet flats were not a great idea," she giggled, wiggling her soaked toes.

Caleb's lips tilted up at the corners. "Okay?" he asked before looking back at his posse of drowned rats. Despite the weather, a collection of whoops and hollers greeted him in reply.

Caleb drove carefully, dropping each person off, making sure they reached their front doors safely before he set off again. He was clearly a good driver, but from the clench of his jaw it was obvious the rain, and the water now rushing the roads, were setting him on edge.

He finally pulled up outside Grace's house and turned off the cruiser. The rain thundered against the roof, hood, and windshield. He looked at her pulling an *eek* face. "On the count of three?"

"One. Two. Three!"

They both darted out of the car, ducking and weaving through the torrents, shouting until they reached the porch. Grace slid the key in the door and pushed, slipping on the laminate floor. Caleb caught her, his hands on her waist for a brief moment, before reaching for the light switch. It clicked but no light appeared.

"Oh no," Grace grumbled, trying it herself, twice.

Caleb shut the door behind him. "Shit. This might have affected the whole town." He frowned at the unresponsive spotlights as though they were somehow to blame. "Where's your fuse box?" he asked, pulling his flashlight from his belt.

Grace laughed nervously. Other than Max and Kai, both of whom she trusted implicitly, she'd not been alone with a man in the house. She moved backward slowly, toward the couch. "Um, I have no idea."

Caleb narrowed his eyes gently, watching her distance. He lifted a hand as though calming a startled animal. "Hey, I just want to make sure you've got power before I leave you, okay?" He un-clipped his radio, holding it out to her. "Do you want to call some-one to come over while I'm here?" His face was entirely indulgent, with no hint of a lie or ulterior motive.

Grace fisted her hands together at her stomach, as the storm battled overhead. "No," she said finally. "Sorry." She waved a dis-missive hand. "I'm just being— Forgive me; it's the storm making me jumpy."

Caleb smiled small. "No worries. I get it." He reattached his radio and turned on his flashlight, as he cleared his throat. "Let's find that fuse box, huh?"

• • • •

After an hour's search, Caleb managed to locate Grace's fuse box and had the power back on before he left. Apparently, despite the extensive work that had taken place, her house's electrics were still touchy about thunder and lightning. Caleb had left soon after and was, as always, polite and gracious. Grace couldn't deny that she felt a tad silly for reacting the way she had with him, but, as Nina had explained, even though she was making positive steps with men in some ways, in others it would still take time.

By noon the following day, the rain had eased and the cracks of thunder had lessened to sporadic rumbles that rolled up and over the mountains. The storm had eased for the most part the horrendous humidity that had smothered the town for days, and Grace didn't hesitate in throwing on her running gear and setting off toward the cottage, along the well-worn track she and Max took daily, and back into town to grab her latte and muffin. The forecast for the evening was much the same, so Grace wasn't planning to dally about.

"Hey, Grace!" Ruby stood at her shop door waving and smil-ing. "Good to see you survived last night."

Grace jogged over, sidestepping the huge puddles that had gathered. "Just. You?"

"Yeah, I'm just checking that my business is still here and hasn't floated away." She laughed.

Grace smiled. "Hey, did your power go out?" Ruby shook her head. "Mine did. Caleb had to fix it."

"Lord. I'm glad he was there to help. Was Max not around?"

Grace frowned. "He's in Philly."

Ruby's smile faltered. "No, they . . . they got back last night. Maybe eight o'clock. Did Max not call? Josh said they decided to risk the weather and head back. I'm glad they did. It was so nice having him in bed last night. I hate storms."

Grace exhaled, a strange, heavy sensation twisting up her back. "I didn't know." She shooed the feeling away with a roll of her shoulders. "He was probably exhausted. I'll call him later." Her eyes found the sky. "Before the next heavyweight bout."

She said her good-byes, called in at the coffee shop, buying Max's regular order as well as her own, and set off toward the boardinghouse. Excitement swelled in her stomach as she climbed the stairs and wandered down the hallway to his door. She knocked twice, hearing him call out before his heavy footsteps approached. She smiled when the lock slid back and it grew as the door opened and revealed him. He was bare-chested, in a pair of worn jeans with nothing on his feet. His hair was chaotic and he hadn't shaved in at least a few days. He was beautiful.

"Hey!" Grace tried her best to curtail her happiness at seeing him, but her high-pitched voice gave her away. "Welcome back." She lifted her offerings to him and it was then that she noticed his expression.

His eyes were so dark they looked flat black. The warm Hershey's Kiss she loved so much was but a faint memory against the intense obsidian glare that greeted her. A muscle in his jaw ticked, while his lips pressed into a flat line that she'd only seen once before: the night he'd gotten drunk at Whiskey's.

She dropped her hands slowly, her smile with it. "You okay?"

His Adam's apple bobbed when he swallowed. "Fine."

The word was curt, cold, and made Grace flinch. Her stare flittered around his face, trying to see past his anger. And he *was* angry; it surged off him. "You don't seem okay."

He huffed a laugh that reeked of sarcasm and rubbed a hand across his chin. His other gripped the door handle so hard his knuckles whitened. "What do you want?"

Grace's breath caught. He'd never spoken to her that way before. "What do you mean?"

"I mean, what do you want? Why are you here?" His nostrils flared and his stare flashed heatedly.

Grace was mystified. "I'm here because . . . I wanted to see you and . . . give you these. I'd have come sooner but I didn't know you were back."

"Yeah, I know."

Annoyance and confusion pushed her words out. "What's wrong with you? What happened?"

Max sighed heavily and glared at a point over her head. "Nothin'. Look, I've got shit to do. I'll see you around, okay?"

"Max, wait." Her plea was met with the sound of the door slamming shut. She knocked again, her knuckles smarting with the force, and called his name twice, but there was no reply. "What the hell?" She remained standing in the hallway, lost and perplexed for what felt like hours before she left his coffee and muffin at the door and made her way back home, where she clambered into bed and tried her damnedest not to cry.

26

Grace rolled over in bed as lightning filled the room. The rain was still falling heavily, the sound like pebbles smacking the window, while the sky continued to complain and snarl every few minutes, as though it were as pissed-off as she was. It was warm again; that horrid, sticky warm that makes fabric stick to your skin like Velcro, and Grace suspected the worst of it was yet to come. She'd been awake for a while, tossing and turning with every bump of the clouds, with Max's irate face flashing behind her eyelids.

She had no idea why he'd behaved so dismissively, said such hurtful things, or why he'd looked at her with such disdain, when all she could think about was launching herself into his arms and begging for him to never let her go. Whatever it was, she was going to get to the bottom of it if it killed her.

She'd texted him twice asking him to talk to her, but he'd yet to reply. The gray dots stayed maddeningly invisible, despite her knowing that he had read each one she'd sent. He was purpose-fully ignoring her and it cut her to the quick. She'd put so much trust into what they had between them so quickly that to have it snatched away with no reason at all left Grace breathless. Never would she have expected him to treat her that way after what he'd been through, after knowing what *she'd* been through. It was cruel and made Grace feel decidedly ill.

"Idiot," she whispered to the empty room. The sky grumbled in agreement.

Lifting her head from her pillow, Grace looked toward her bedroom door, cocking her head. She was almost certain she'd heard a noise, or a knock of some kind, maybe the jangle of a key. Pausing from a brief moment, she reached out and flicked on her bedside light, almost crippled in relief when it turned on, shooing the darkness away.

A floorboard creaked.

"Oh God." Paralyzed, Grace widened her eyes as the door handle on her bedroom door turned. She knew she kept a baseball bat under the bed—there was even a gun in the safe that Kai had given her—but she couldn't move.

"Don't," she managed, her voice surprisingly firm. "I have a gun. I have a gu—"

"It's me." Grace's heart nearly collapsed in her chest, as the door opened and Max appeared, sopping wet, her key hider in his open palm. "Don't shoot."

"Jesus Christ!" Grace yelled, kneeling up quickly and pelting him with one, two, three of her scatter cushions, launching them across the room, hitting him square in the face with the first. "You scared me to death! What the hell were you thinking?"

He held his arms up to block any more potential missiles. "I was thinking I needed to talk to you."

"At two a.m.?"

"Yeah, at fucking two a.m. I couldn't sleep." His tone was sharp, the remnants of whatever had him so out of shape still clutching every word. He stood up straight, when the last cushion hit the floor, staring hard at her. Ordinarily, Grace would have shrunk back at his attempts at intimidation, but the adrenaline had kicked in, and she wasn't backing down.

She looked him up and down, noticing that the running shoes and his sweatpants up to the knee were drenched and caked in mud.

"You ran here?" she exclaimed, glancing toward the window.

"Yeah, so?" he retorted defensively. "I think better when I run."

Yeah, Grace knew that. He'd told her so before. "So." She gestured toward him with a wave of her hand. "Are you here to tell me what the hell is wrong with you and why you acted like such an ass today?"

Max inhaled through his nose, his large shoulders lifting. Grace noticed he did this when he was trying to rein in his temper. He rubbed the bridge of his nose and shook his head. "You're unbelievable," he muttered toward his shoes.

"*I* am?" Grace countered loudly. "You're the one who slammed the door in my face."

Max's head snapped up, surprise flickering over his features before he quickly schooled them. "Look, I came here to say what I needed to say and then I'm out of here, all right?"

Grace crossed her arms over her chest, still kneeling in the center of her bed. "Fine."

He pointed toward the floor between them, rainwater falling to the carpet. "I know I'm an asshole, okay, and I know us sleeping together was never going to be straightforward. I get that. But, whatever. I decided I'd be exclusive to you because that's what you deserved." His voice dropped in volume. "I know I never asked for you to do the same because, one, I didn't expect you'd be flashing your shit to anyone else and two, it ain't got nothing to do with me." His rising anger caused his Brooklyn twang to grow stronger. "But I didn't expect you to treat me like a fucking fool. I ain't one and I *don't* deserve that."

"Max." Grace breathed deeply in an effort to calm herself. "I have no idea what you're talking about."

He stepped back, looking toward his feet. "I saw you, Grace." He lifted his head and for the first time, Grace detected hurt. "I saw you with him." He licked his lips and glanced toward the ceiling, pressing his lips together. "I saw you laughing . . . he touched you and you were both in here— Look, whatever, it's fine." He ran his hands through his wet hair and mumbled something toward the wall. "I would have rather you just told me before fucking around with that prick."

Grace regarded him carefully as all the pieces started to fall into place. There was only one person she knew who got Max as riled as this, one person he referred to with such aggression.

"You saw me with Caleb."

He coughed a noise that was no doubt a curse, despite the wounded glint she caught in his gaze. "Bingo."

Grace unfolded her arms, her body heavy with fatigue and disappointment. "You saw me with Caleb," she repeated. "And you think what? That I slept with him?" He didn't answer except to cock an eyebrow, the challenge clear. Her heart squeezed. She dropped her chin to her chest and tried to gather herself. "You know what, Max? You're right." She looked back at him. "You *are* an asshole."

Max's head moved back as though he'd been slapped. "Say what, now?"

Grace shook her head and drew back the sheet so she could climb under. "Please lock the door when you leave."

"Are you kidding me?" His voice lifted at the end, causing Grace to turn.

"No. I'm not," she replied, calm and monotone.

Max scowled with his arms out wide. "And that's it. No denial, no explanation, nothing?"

Grace shook her head slowly. The only denial she could see was his. "You saw what you wanted to see, Max, nothing more. I could spend the next hour explaining what was actually happening, and why, but it wouldn't matter."

"Why wouldn't it matter?" he snapped.

Grace's heart thumped at the fire in his eyes. He was too stubborn to realize what he was feeling, too blind to see what was right in front of him, but it wasn't the time to try to show him. As much as it pained Grace, she knew he'd have to come to the realization on his own. "Would it matter to you, Max?"

"Yes!"

"Why?" She spoke so softly and he was silent for so long, Grace wondered whether he'd heard her.

The moment was broken when thunder cracked above them, making the lights dim. Rain pummeled the roof, getting harder and more aggressive as the seconds passed. Max stared at Grace, still without voice, though, she noted, the warm brown tones of his eyes had started to creep back and the softness that she loved so much about his face smoothed the angry lines that had creased it.

Relieved, she nodded toward him. "Get undressed and get in here."

He blinked, his eyebrows meeting above his nose. "What?"

"You're soaked and it's like the apocalypse out there. You're not driving and you sure as hell aren't walking, so get in here until it passes." She didn't wait for him to reply and continued getting under the thin sheet, her back to him. He didn't move. Grace squeezed her eyes shut. "Max. Please."

"I shouldn't."

"I know." She took a deep breath. "But I don't want you to go."

There was another stretch of quiet before the unmistakable rustle of clothes being removed could be heard. He padded around her room, placing his clothes on the radiator and his wallet and keys on the nightstand next to her, and eventually crawled into bed.

"Thank you," she whispered, her shoulders dropping with the sensation of having him so close, as though his mere presence helped her breathe easier.

"Just until it passes," he replied, his voice gruff, but quiet.

She reached out to turn off the lamp. "Okay."

.   .   .

It was before dawn when Grace woke again. It was still dark. The thunder had eased but still the rain came. Grace nuzzled the pillow and sighed. While they slept, Max had moved closer, his body molding around hers, his hand tentative on her hip. He'd done this before when they'd fallen asleep together despite claiming that he wasn't one for hugs or spooning. He was full of it, though; the man was made for snuggling.

In spite of their heated words, Grace smiled when his breath washed against her neck. He felt so good behind her that she was unable to resist shifting back in an effort to feel more of him. It had been too long since she'd felt so safe. Surely, he was feeling what she was, right? The expanding that occurred in her chest every time she saw him, the butterflies when he smiled, the insane lust when they came together. It had to be real.

"Quit moving," he grumbled sleepily, his nose pressing into the skin behind her ear.

It was on her next breath to ask why, but the way his hips flexed against her ass told her loud and clear why his words sounded tight. Wow. The way he was so blatant about how his body reacted to hers never failed to make Grace warm all over. Life would be so much simpler if he could be so open with his heart.

"Sorry."

"No you're not," he retorted, calling her out at the same time she pushed against him again. He huffed a breath. "Don't start what you can't finish."

Grace was struck with how perfectly those words fit their relationship. Their argument had done nothing but underline just how fragile they still both were, while the overwhelming feeling that, inevitably, they were headed for a serious conversation filled Grace with resounding fear. She didn't want to lose him. She couldn't.

"Max." His name slipped between her lips before she could stop it and she placed her hand on the back of his as it traveled up her waist and back down to the top of her thigh.

"What do you want?" he asked, his tongue flicking out to taste her skin.

She swallowed back the many things she wanted from him, for him, for them, and said simply, "You."

His fingers dipped teasingly to her inner thigh at the same time he pushed his erection against her ass. "Just me?"

She turned her head sharply at the unspoken insinuation of his question. Meeting his tired yet hopeful eyes, however, made the angry response curl back heavily into her chest. She was so exhausted hiding what she felt for him, what she wanted with him. She could only be honest and hope that, in time, he would return the favor. "It's always been just you. Nothing happened with Caleb, Max. He got my lights working again and left. I swear to you."

He closed his eyes briefly, as though her words were exactly what he needed to hear, and slipped his hand swiftly between her legs and under the elastic of her sleep shorts. Grace arched when his fingers found her. They played her perfectly, firm but teasing, fast then slow, dipping and rubbing her in ways that had her calling out nonsense, clutching his forearm just to feel the muscles as they worked her.

"Yes," she breathed. "Please."

He slipped two fingers into her, curling them to stroke her in places that made her call out his name.

"Who?" he growled in her ear, his hips undulating against her, while his hand began to move faster, his fingers fucking her so perfectly.

"You, Max," she groaned. "Don't stop."

"Wallet," he grunted into her shoulder.

Holding back her moans, and with his fingers continuing to pull pleasure from her very bones, Grace reached over for his wallet and quickly pulled out the two condoms she knew would be there. Throwing the wallet back on the nightstand, she held one of the condoms out to him. He opened his mouth and took it between his teeth.

"Come," he grit out around it. "I know you're close."

He wasn't wrong. He knew her body as well as she did. She

groaned and nodded, relaxing herself from head to toe, allowing him to bring her to a climax that was sharp, loud, and altogether incredible. He shushed and soothed her, his palm stroking her between her legs until she was shivering in his arms.

"It's all right. I've got you," he told her, pulling back slightly to remove his underwear.

Grace rid herself of her cami and shorts and watched over her shoulder, entranced, as he rolled on the condom. He was just so damned gorgeous to look at. He glanced up at her, waiting, as he always did for her to tell him that she was fine for him to start. She smiled gently, gaining one in reply. He lifted her thigh and ducked his head, kissing her shoulder blade softly as he pushed into her from behind.

That feeling. That feeling right there where they joined was something Grace could never explain. He filled her, yes, but it was more than that. It was as if, when he pushed his body into hers, her soul exhaled in relief, as though it had finally found what it had been searching for for so long.

He drew back his hips and pushed back, pushing a moan from Grace's throat. He clutched her to him, his hands on her breasts, his mouth right by her ear. "He wants this," he said, anger teasing the words. "He wants you just like this."

Knowing "he" was Caleb, Grace moved her hand to the back of Max's head, over her shoulder, and gripped his hair. "He can't have me like this," she told him. "He's never had me like this. He'll *never* have me like this."

He mumbled her name into her neck. "Why? Tell me why, Gracie."

She turned to look at him, struggling with the angle. "Because only you have me like this."

The sound that came from Max's throat was unconcealed possessiveness that lifted the very hairs on Grace's arms. He thrust firmly, growling and holding her so hard his fingers pinched.

"Wait," she gasped. "Max, wait."

He slowed, his hips still rolling, but his voice panicked. "Was I too rough?"

"No."

"What is it?"

"I want to see you."

He didn't hesitate. He pulled away and lay on his back waiting for her to ride him.

"No," she said, pushing her unease away as her gaze prowled down his magnificent body. "I want you on top this time."

There was a flash of surprise with a hint of uncertainty across Max's face before he nodded. "If you're sure."

"Absolutely." And she was. She trusted the man climbing over her and settling between her legs more than any other man she'd ever been with, and whether he'd admit it or not, she knew that he cared for her enough to never harm her. Max's placed his hands at either side of her shoulders, still careful not to put any weight on her.

"Put me in you." His request, said, as always, in that unintentionally erotic way of his, turned Grace's bones to mush.

She put her hand around his cock and guided him. He slipped in perfectly as he always did, only this time she could wrap her legs around his waist. In doing so, she brought his weight onto her. Her breath faltered, panic teasing at the edges of her psyche, making Max pause. "I'm okay," she urged. "Honestly."

Long-lashed Hershey's Kisses roamed over her face until, seemingly satisfied with what he saw, Max began moving again, breathing heavily, eyes closing, then opening, then rolling back while his lips twitched and pursed whenever his teeth weren't worrying them. Seeing the muscles in his shoulders bunch and his neck cord was hypnotizing. He was sublime. Their eyes met and he groaned, dropping his weight to his forearms, and his face to her throat.

"You feel so good," he said, lifting her thigh farther up his hip and shoving hard into her.

He hissed and lifted his face to her jaw. His stubble rubbed her as he moved over and over, hot and eager. He felt divine. He wound his hips in a tantalizing figure eight, pushing into her farther.

"I want to make you come again," he moaned. "I want to feel it on my cock."

Grace's eyes rolled back at his commanding tone. "Oh God."

She whimpered as they rocked together, sopping and hot. The sensation of him moving inside her made it impossible to think, let alone move or form words. She was beyond coherence, and it was sublime.

I love you.

"There," she gasped as he hit one particularly toe-curling spot.

He did it again and began to move faster. Grace gripped his shoulders and groaned as her stomach began to tighten. Her thighs held his securely and her back arched.

"You feel so fucking good," Max panted. He pushed his hips up so quickly that Grace's lifted from the bed. "Can you feel how hard you make me?"

She hummed into his cheek. Max looked down at where their bodies were writhing together. His brow furrowed and his lips pursed. "Holy shit, Gracie."

She moved again, grinding down in a circular motion, making Max grip her waist. Grace threw her arms around his neck and buried her nose into his hair, inhaling, taking every breath of scent he had to offer.

"I missed you," she said. "I missed you so much."

He lifted his head, inches away. He didn't speak, but his face told her that her words, although surprising, were welcome.

"I did," she affirmed. "I thought about you like you asked."

He grunted again and thrust, making Grace's neck elongate, while sporadic moans left him with each drive of his hips. He was so close, his body, his face, his lips, and, without thinking, Grace lifted her mouth to meet his in a desperate kiss.

His reaction was immediate.

He froze, pulling away as though she'd burned him. "Don't!"

"I'm sorry," she exclaimed, genuinely stunned by her own actions, while also relieved he hadn't removed himself from her body. "God, I'm so sorry."

Max lifted a hand and thumped it back down onto the bed next to her face. "Dammit, Grace."

"I didn't mean to—I don't even—I just . . ."

He swallowed, watching her carefully, jaw clenching. "Just what?"

She forced herself to meet his gaze. "I'm sorry." Her hand moved from his waist to his ass. "Truly. I wasn't thinking. Please. Don't stop."

He paused for a moment and then, with a sigh that sounded like he had little choice in the matter, he did as she asked.

Grace hissed when he tilted his hips and hit her just right. "Yes, like that." He hummed, his stare intense, cracking her verbal filter into a thousand pieces. "I love you inside me. I missed this. Harder."

Her nails trailed down his back, squeezing his ass as he sped up, making his strokes deeper, sharper. He moaned. "Fuck."

"I want you like this all the time, Max," Grace confessed, the roll of his hips between her thighs beyond perfect.

"Tell me."

"All the time. I *think* about it all the time."

"How?"

"I imagine it . . . I touched myself, you know? Like you asked. I did. I couldn't help it. I—"

Her words came to an abrupt halt, eaten up by Max's ravenous mouth as he kissed her.

Grace flailed under the unexpected pressure of his lips, his unshaven face deliciously rough, and the air plummeting out his nose against her cheek. Gathering herself, she returned his kiss with all the passion and heat she'd hidden since she'd met him. She gripped his hair, pulling him impossibly closer. He growled and pushed his tongue into her mouth, seeking out hers and sucking it. At the same time, he shoved into her harder and harder, skin slapping beautifully, bed creaking, and Grace's muffled cries rising in volume. His lips chased hers, nibbling and biting, sloppy and desperate, as if he'd been as starved as she was for it, until, with one final thrust, he pulled his head back and roared toward the ceiling, coming with such force, his hips lifted Grace from the bed.

Eyes squeezed shut, he moaned with each exhale and twitch of his cock in her, finally collapsing onto Grace, his head burrowed under her chin, panting against her collarbone. Welcoming his weight, she wrapped herself around him, clinging to him with every part of herself and kissing his hair as his body vibrated with aftershocks.

"I've got you," she whispered, her lips against his forehead. "I promise. I've got you."

He shuddered, his breaths heavy and shaky, and when he spoke, it was through a thick, overwhelmed throat. "Wh-what are you doing to me?"

Grace closed her eyes and stroked the side of his face. "What does it feel like?"

He shivered. "Terrifying."

Grace's heartbeat tripped over itself. Gradually, Max lifted his head. The brown of his eyes shimmered with unshed emotion. She cupped his face and leaned up to kiss him again. There was a hint of hesitation before he returned it gently, the tremor in his body prevalent.

"Don't be scared," she told him as she rubbed the side of her nose against his. "Not of me. I only want to love you."

His face collapsed as though it was the worst news he'd ever heard. "Don't," he begged. "Gracie, don't. Please."

She smiled a melancholy smile before she stole another kiss. "Too late."

She was surprised that he didn't argue. He simply pulled out of her and laid his head on her chest. Although his silence was better than the row she was positive was coming, it still made her decidedly uneasy. She was proud that she'd been so brave, so honest and open with him, and the relief that seized her was as exhilarating as it was welcome. Max lifted himself from the bed and cleaned up, shocking the hell out of her when, instead of dressing and leaving as he normally did, he crawled back in, snuggling up and holding her closely.

She was even more surprised when, a few hours later, he woke her to make love again. It was heartbreakingly slow and tender, just like the kisses they shared, his voice hoarse with emotion as he talked her through her orgasm, holding her face in his hands, before calling out into her mouth when his followed soon after. It was beautiful and perfect, which made it hurt even more when she awoke again, just before noon, to find his side of the bed empty, with no sign that he was ever there at all.

27

His time in rehab notwithstanding, Max was more than aware of the stupid shit he'd done in his life. He'd fucked people over, treated them like crap, made impulsive decisions that always came back to bite him, and threw people under the bus with no regret, always making sure that he was the one who came out untarnished when shit hit the fan, no matter who got hurt. Yeah, he was a prize asshole, but that shit wasn't news. What *was* news and what really had his brain on fast spin while he lay on his bed in the boarding-house, his body aching in all the ways it should after a night of incredible sex and very little sleep, was that Max knew he'd finally outdone himself.

Last night.

Shit. Last night.

What had happened between him and Grace had been . . .

He exhaled.

It had been amazing.

Plain and simple. There was no point in denying it. Sex with her always was and last night was no exception.

Christ, he'd been livid on Friday after stumbling upon her and the asshole cop laughing and touching as they went into her house, and he'd had every intention of calling the whole thing off. Standing in the pounding rain, hidden by the trees and watching them like some cheap film cliché, he'd realized he wasn't prepared to share Grace with anyone, least of all that dick-with-a-badge deputy. He'd run back to her house at 2 a.m. to tell her just that, letting the storm stir his fury further, grumbling to himself about what a stupid decision it was to get involved with anyone, and promising himself that he was going to stay away from women indefinitely to avoid the stress of it all.

Nevertheless, as determined as he had been, somewhere along the line Max's plan had dissolved into oblivion. It may have had something to do with how hot it was seeing Grace fired up, standing tall, not being intimidated by him, and, strangely, Max couldn't help but feel that in some small way, he was responsible for the confidence she had to go toe-to-toe with him. Her fire was sexy as hell and when her eyes flashed, challenging him and his accusation, he knew he was fucked.

Of course she hadn't gone to bed with the prick. Deep down Max had known that all along, stubbornly refusing to investigate why he'd assumed such a thing in the first place. Was it jealousy? Was he so involved with Grace now that jealousy factored in to it? He couldn't tell, but he knew that seeing that piece of shit put his hands on her had made Max seriously consider homicide.

And then there was the kiss.

He rubbed his hands down his face, trying his damnedest not to think about the taste of her lips, her eager mouth, and her passionate tongue, which lapped at him as if he were some kind of precious elixir or something. He'd promised himself not to let anyone get that close, but hearing her words, her begging, her pleading, her dirty mutterings, after being teased by her impulsive kiss, it was all too much for him to take. The urge to have more had risen through him like a tidal wave. He'd been so fucking foolish to let that happen. Kissing blurred things, created feelings, and that was a minefield Max had no intention of navigating again. And he hadn't, not for a long time.

He'd not kissed a woman like that since . . . Lizzie, and even then, he struggled to pull to memory a time where the two of them had been that frantic to taste one another. He'd come to the conclusion that, somehow, that was different. He'd loved Lizzie, spent years with her where, over time, as was the case in most relationships, their passion and need for each other morphed from explosive flash-bang fireworks into something quieter, calmer, but no less hot.

"Fuck," he muttered toward the ceiling. He had no idea what his next step was. He'd crept out of Grace's bed, avoiding looking at her so warm and beautiful as she slept, and left the house like the coward he was. He didn't even leave a note, but then, what the hell would he have written? His head was a hot mess, and until he decided what he was going to do, he needed to stay away from her.

It was almost too much for him, an addict, to cope with. His cravings, for the most part, stayed relatively quiet, but that could all change if he didn't sort his shit out. His eight-month NA coin dipped and flicked between the knuckles of his right hand. Thank God for his anti-anxiety meds, he thought wryly. He closed his eyes, trying to breathe deeply, but a knock at the door had them snapping back open.

Panic seized him.

Grace.

What the hell would he say to her? He'd already beaten himself up for slamming the door in her face once, he couldn't do that again, but he didn't have any answers to the questions she'd have and deserved to ask. The knock came again, firmer and not sounding at all like the polite, timid knock that Grace always gave. Max cleared his throat and heaved himself off the bed, approaching the door and resting his forehead against it for a brief moment, trying to gather what courage he could to face whatever was standing on the other side.

Holding his breath, he unlocked it and swung it open. "Carter!"

He was so surprised to see his friend, and even more relieved to find him and not Grace standing there, that he was unable to keep himself from pulling his buddy in for a huge hug, slapping his back and smiling.

Stumbling into the embrace, Carter hugged him back. That was reassuring; at least he wasn't there to deliver bad news.

"What the hell, man?" Max asked. "What are you doing here?" He stood back, clasping Carter's shoulders. He looked okay, dressed casual in a gray Henley, dark blue jeans, and a beat-up brown light-weight motorcycle jacket. It looked to be more for fashion than function, but it was still badass.

"I thought I'd come and see you," Carter grinned. "You know, see how you're doin'."

Max narrowed his eyes. "Bullshit. You're here hiding from Kat, aren't you?"

Carter snorted, rubbing a palm across the back of his neck. "Maybe."

Max waved a hand. "Well, whatever, come in." He stood back for Carter to enter and closed the door behind him. It was so good to see his best friend, especially in light of the fact that shit was not at all copacetic. Maybe a little normalcy was what Max needed to pull his head out of his ass.

With his hands in the pockets of his jeans, Carter looked around the room, his gaze spending time on the canvases in the corner of the room. He approached them and dropped to his haunches as he took a closer look. Carter's finger moved over the lime-green patterns of one particular piece. "These are great," he commented.

"They're all right," Max muttered, reaching to grab a pair of worn blue jeans to change into. He'd been slopping in sweats since his shower after he arrived back at the boardinghouse that morning.

"Modesty doesn't suit you," Carter said over his shoulder. "This one would look sweet in my apartment."

"Then take it," Max uttered dismissively. He wasn't fond of the green anyway.

Still crouched, Carter turned at the waist. "Really?"

"Call it a birthday gift."

"My birthday was in March." Carter smirked.

"Shit, really?" Max paused. "Then it's a belated birthday gift. Surprise!"

Carter laughed, shaking his head. "Thanks."

After a silent moment where Carter's stare on him began to make Max nervous, Carter stood and wandered closer. "You okay?"

Max ran a hand through his hair, debating quickly whether to simply spill. He settled for giving a lackadaisical shrug. "Sure."

Carter tilted his head in the way that Max recognized. He was looking for a lie. "Well, you look good, dude. The West Virginia air is working its magic, huh?"

Max coughed an uneasy laugh. "Yeah, look, what do you say we go and get some coffee?"

"Food, too. I'm starving. Haven't eaten since breakfast."

"You drove?"

"From the airport." Carter grimaced at Max's questioning frown. "Company private jet."

"Shit, man."

"I know," Carter said with a shrug. "But it was that or drive for four hours and I need to head back tonight."

Max nodded as he grabbed his keys and wallet. "Flying visit then."

"Seems that way." Carter walked out in front of Max and waited as he locked up. "So how are things?"

Max pocketed his keys and walked shoulder to shoulder with Carter down the hallway toward the stairs of the boardinghouse. "I'm . . . okay." Carter didn't look convinced, lifting a curious eyebrow, which Max tried to ignore. "It's nothing major. I'm just a fucking idiot."

Carter snorted. "That's not news, man."

Max laughed as they reached the foot of the stairs and pulled the boardinghouse door open to let Carter through. A fast-moving body who exclaimed, "I'm so sorry," careened into him.

Max gripped soft arms, smelled cocoa butter, and immediately let go, stepping back. "Grace," he blurted.

Christ, it was just like the first time they'd met, she bumping into him, all nervous and flustered. Except now she didn't look flustered. She looked tired and unhappy. She gazed up at him, her green eyes expectant, but Max had no words of comfort for her. He had no words at all. The silence in the small vestibule became suffocating, before she glanced over to Carter, who smiled and held out his hand.

"I'll introduce myself, shall I?" he said, knocking his shoulder against Max's. "Carter."

They shook hands and Max watched a perfect smile crease Grace's face.

"Max's best friend," she said. "I've heard a lot about you."

"None of it's true," Carter replied. "Well, some of it. Okay. Maybe all of it."

Grace gave a little laugh at the same time Max shifted on his feet. Carter looked back and forth between the two of them, noticing the tension. Jesus, Max could barely look at her. Not that he didn't want to; she was gorgeous. But the shame that clutched his chest, along with something that was both heavy and foreign, kept his eyes stuck resolutely to the floor. He wanted nothing more than for that sucker to swallow him whole.

"We're just heading for a late lunch," Carter added. "Do you wanna come?"

Max threw him a look that would have rendered any other man dead on the spot. "No," he said before Grace could answer. "She has stuff to do." He finally looked at her. "Don't you?"

Guilt and frustration burned up his back when he saw the wounded flicker in her eyes. "Sure." She took a deep breath and looked to Carter. "Sure. You two have fun. It was nice to meet you." She pinned Max with a look that defied argument. "I'll talk to you later."

Max nodded. It wasn't until the door closed behind her that he felt he could breathe.

Carter whistled low. "Dude, what the fuck was that?"

Max rubbed his temples with the pads of his fingers. "I can't— It's not what you think. It's not what it looks like."

Carter smirked, seeing through Max's lie. "Really? Because from your face I think it's exactly what it looks like." He glanced toward the door as though he could still see Grace through it. "Why the hell haven't you mentioned her before?"

Wasn't that the million-dollar question? Max lifted his shoulders toward his ears, opening his mouth to say something, but nothing came. He exhaled on a growl and yanked the door open. "I'll tell you everything over a strong coffee."

So he did. Sitting in his usual seat in the quiet coffee shop, Max relayed the last four months to his best friend, every moment between him and Grace, her past, the arrangement they made, July Fourth, the cellar, up to and including the night before. Carter sat quietly, occasionally sipping his espresso. He didn't ask questions and never looked judgmental. Max could have hugged him again for it. Truthfully, it felt good to purge.

Thumping back in his seat, Max waited for Carter to hit him with a glorious piece of advice. Instead, he sighed and ran his index finger around the rim of his cup.

He seemed to mull over what he was going to say until Max couldn't take it anymore. "Spit it out, please," he complained.

Carter frowned. "I'm not sure you wanna hear what I think."

Max placed his elbows on the table and dropped his chin into his hands. "No, man, I really do." He cupped his fingers over his mouth, waiting. "I . . . I'm at a loss here."

Carter sat forward, mirroring Max's pose. "My first question is, why? Why start this?"

Max had asked himself the same thing, and the only answer he could come up with was why the hell not. He said as much to Carter, who appeared uncomfortable with the answer. "That's a shitty reason."

Max nodded in agreement, but there it was.

"I have to ask," Carter said quietly. "Is this just about sex?" Max opened his mouth to reply, but Carter stopped him. "What I mean is, she seems like a nice girl, beautiful. I mean, she trusted you enough, right? Could it be more? Is that why you're freaking out?"

Max paused for a moment, mulling that over. "I like her," he admitted through his fingers. "But, no. It's not anything more."

Carter's eyes narrowed infinitesimally. "Do you want it to be?"

Max dropped his hands back to the tabletop and shook his head. "I can't, man. You know that."

"Lizzie," Carter said as though the mere thought of her offended him. "That woman . . ."

"Don't. It's not worth it."

"Yeah, but *you* are," Carter snapped. "I wish you'd see that." He rubbed a hand across his forehead wearily. "You're worth it, Max. You're worth— You're worth more than her, more than her coming into your life, turning it upside down, and fuckin' leaving you with no word, no care, to slowly kill yourself."

Max sat back, frowning at his best friend. "Wow."

Carter had been understandably vocal in his hatred of Lizzie before, but this was something else. "Where the hell did that come from?" Max asked.

Carter blew out a heavy breath and dragged his bottom teeth across his top lip. He glared at his coffee cup and Max watched as his friend tried to gather himself. "I hate what she did to you," Carter snarled quietly.

"I know," Max replied, his voice softened with Carter's concern. "Me, too."

"Tell me something." Carter looked up slowly. "What would you say to her if you ever saw her again?"

Max had allowed himself a million fleeting moments to wonder about that and he was still without an answer. He lifted a shoulder. "I don't know."

"Would you even want to see her?"

Something in Carter's voice made the hair on Max's neck lift. He cocked his head, trying to see in Carter's eyes what he was hiding.

"Why?" He frowned. "It's not like that's a possibility now, is it?"

Carter didn't answer. He merely stared back across the table, his blue eyes guarded.

"Carter?" Max sat forward. "What's going on?"

After a brief moment where Carter seemed to come to some sort of decision, he licked his lips and looked out of the coffee shop window to the wet street outside. He reached into the inside pocket of his biker jacket and pulled out a creased white envelope. He stared at it for a beat, gave an aggrieved sigh, and placed it on the table before sliding it across to Max.

"*This* is why I'm here. It arrived two days ago."

Max stared at the envelope with his name and address on the front of it, noting the cursive patterns of the handwriting. He'd know that fucking penmanship anywhere. *Lizzie.* His heart skipped an entire beat, as the realization rushed over him like a bucket of ice water, forcing Max back in his seat with a harsh exhalation. He lifted his hands as though the mere thought of touching the envelope filled him with terror.

"I wanted to give it to you in person instead of forwarding it on to you like I do your bills."

Max swallowed, not entirely certain whether he was going to throw up or pass out. His head swam horrifically. "Ha-have you read it?" He noticed that the flap of the envelope was ripped.

"I open all your mail, like you asked me to, but I had no idea who it was from until I read the first few lines and saw the name at the bottom."

Carter ran his hands across his short hair, appearing truly torn with his having to give the letter over.

The two men sat in silence, both looking at the damned thing as though it might explode. Max shoved his thumbnail into his mouth and started chewing. It was an anxious gesture he'd not indulged in since he'd left rehab.

"What—why . . ." he mumbled around his thumb, looking at Carter helplessly. "What do I do?"

Carter's brow creased in sympathy, his gaze worried. "That's up to you, brother." He pressed his lips together. "You gonna read it?"

The squeeze in Max's chest suggested not, but the curiosity was too much to ignore. Terrified or not, Max knew that he would be reading the fucking thing one way or another.

His face must have answered Carter, who dipped his head in understanding. "You want me to stay here while you do?"

As much as Max appreciated the offer, he knew he had to face whatever that letter contained on his own. "No," he croaked.

Carter nodded. "Go take a walk, okay? Maybe call Tate. Get some space."

The air in the shop had certainly grown stuffy; Max could barely catch his breath. He allowed his finger to trace his name on the envelope. Carter's hand on his shoulder made him jump. Max hadn't even noticed him stand.

"I'll go and hang at the bar down the street," he said, his eyes drifting to the letter. "Come when you're ready and we'll talk, okay?"

Max nodded and pushed his chair back, struggling to make his legs hold his weight as he stood. Carter gripped Max's bicep to hold him steady, waited a beat, and pulled him into a tight embrace. Max didn't hesitate in returning it. He wasn't too much of an asshole to admit when he needed a hug. And right then, he needed as many as he could get.

What the hell could Lizzie want after all these years? What could she possibly have to say to him? Why now? He dropped his forehead to Carter's shoulder and breathed deeply, fighting off the petrified tears that threatened.

"I'm here," Carter murmured, cupping the back of Max's head. "You're not alone in this. Whatever you decide, I'll support you."

Max nodded and clapped his hand against Carter's back. "Thank you."

He felt Carter nod before he stepped back. "Text me," he said quietly, and without another word, he left Max in the coffee shop, wondering what the fuck he was going to do.

•   •   •

Grace sat on her sofa, where she'd planted herself three hours before after returning from the boardinghouse. The TV played quietly from its position in the corner of the room, but Grace had no idea what the hell was on it. She was too busy watching the guilt and regret she'd seen so clearly in Max's dark eyes playing like a damn loop in her mind.

Grace hadn't known what to expect when she'd made the decision to seek him out so they could talk, but his curt indifference and coldness certainly weren't anywhere near the top of the list. It had hurt so much seeing his uneasiness, the way he stepped back from her so quickly, his need for the earth to open up under his feet. He couldn't hide that from her; she knew him too well.

She'd spent hours reasoning with herself, trying to understand how terrified Max would be after what they'd shared. Jesus, he'd admitted as much when they were in bed. But even that couldn't soothe the harsh sting of rejection or delete the echo of his words when he'd dismissed her so readily. Could he not see how terrified *she* was? She pulled the throw she'd draped over herself closer. Despite the warm July air, she was cold.

Glancing at the clock to see it was a little before six, she contemplated texting Max. She fingered her cell for the hundredth time, torn between calling her therapist for advice and calling Max. No. Space. That's what he needed. She didn't want to crowd him or make him feel pressured. As she'd told him, all she wanted to do was love him, no titles, no expectations; he'd told her before that he wasn't capable of that, despite the fact that he'd made love to her so tenderly. Grace knew too well that he was a serious flight risk. If she were to ask him for anything more than he was willing to give, he would bolt. She would reserve judgment and do her best to let him mull the whole situation over. She knew that's what he needed. It was what he did.

There was a gentle knock on the front door that Grace considered ignoring. She didn't want to see anyone. It would take only a small question, a sympathetic glance and she'd fall apart. With a sigh, she lifted from the sofa and made her way to the front door.

Max stood on her porch, head down, hands in his jeans pockets, looking as bad as Grace felt. He looked up as she opened the door. Seeing him, hair in disarray, desperate for a shave along with the memory of his body over hers, Grace found her legs suddenly shaky, and leaned subtly against the door's edge for support.

"Hey," she said, her voice small. She glanced at the hidden key spot. "Thanks for knocking."

He swallowed and nodded sharply. His eyes were still wary, still confused and scared, and it broke Grace's heart.

"Do you want to come in?"

He shook his head. "No," he replied quickly, throwing a thumb over his shoulder toward a very flashy-looking car, inside of which was Carter. "I'm not staying."

Grace let the heavy meaning behind his words settle into her. She bit her lip to hold back her panic. "Not staying here"—she pointed toward the floor—"or not staying in Preston County?"

Max's eyes darted to the side before they settled on her again. "Both."

Grace's breath stuttered as it entered her lungs. "Where are you going?"

He licked his lips, looking for a moment as if he intended not to tell her. "Back to New York."

"For good?"

"I don't know, Grace," he growled, looking toward the sky as though asking God for strength. "I'm just . . . shit. I need to go, all right?"

Grace's pulse kicked up, his tone and abrasive attitude no longer hurting but angering her. She didn't deserve it. She'd done nothing but care for him. "Yeah, all right. I mean, it makes sense for you to go."

Max's eyes narrowed suspiciously. "Why?"

"Well, you have always been good at *running*," she commented sharply, arching an eyebrow at him when his shoulders lifted in anger. "What?" she challenged. "You don't think I can see what you're doing?"

Max laughed humorlessly, his eyes flashing dangerously. "You don't see anything. You have no idea."

"Then why don't you explain it to me?" she said bluntly, standing tall, no longer needing the door. "You owe me that much."

His nostrils flared, but she saw the realization of what she said being true wash across his face. He took a deep breath and looked toward his boots, avoiding her pointed look. "Lizzie."

Grace's eyes widened. "Lizzie?"

Max nodded. "Carter brought a letter she wrote me . . ." He lifted his head. He looked so exhausted. "She wants me to meet her. She wants to talk."

Grace was struck dumb. That was the last thing she expected him to say and that changed things. Massively. The fight in her slowly began to ebb away.

With everything that Max had told her about Lizzie and what happened between them, of course it made sense for him to go to her. He would need closure after everything he'd been through. He deserved that. Still, a dark part of Grace couldn't help but wonder if Lizzie's letter was the escape Max needed to get away, to run instead of talking about what had happened the previous night.

Beneath the understanding, cold realization settled in her chest. "So you're meeting her?"

Max rubbed the tips of his fingers across his forehead. "No, I'm not, I— Maybe, I don't even know if I *will*, I just . . ."

Grace swallowed and when she spoke her voice was careful and quiet. "Came here because you want me to tell you it's okay to go."

Max's face creased with incredulity. "What?"

She smiled sadly, resignation slithering through her.

He didn't want her. Not in the way she wanted him. He was too busy clinging to a past to see what was right in front of him and, honestly, she was simply too tired to keep trying to convince him she was right for him.

"I get it, Max, I do," she uttered honestly. "It's important that you two speak. She has a lot to explain, a lot to apologize for. You deserve that."

He frowned, his eyes suspicious. "Yeah, I do."

Grace nodded, pressing her lips together to hold back the desperate words that threatened: *I love you, come back to me, stop running.*

Instead she said, "Will you tell me something before you go?"

Max sighed, glancing back at Carter's car. "Sure."

"Tell me you didn't feel something last night. Tell me it meant nothing to you."

He stared at her for a moment, his jaw ticking. She knew she'd backed him into a corner and he didn't like it, but she had to know he felt what they'd shared. Of course, it made no difference; she was under no illusions that he was leaving no matter what, but at least she'd know that last night was something special for both of them.

"It was what it was," he answered finally, his voice flat. He shrugged belligerently. "A fuck is a fuck, you know?"

Grace's heart stammered as his words hit like bullets. She knew he was lashing out because he was afraid, but they crippled her all the same.

"You don't mean that," she said, her voice wavering.

"I don't?" He shook his head in a way that could only be described as patronizing. "Shit. I knew this was a mistake."

"This?" Grace asked, hating the shake in her knees. She gripped the doorframe.

"You!" Max bit out. "I told you all I wanted was sex," he continued, his voice frustrated, as though he were explaining something simple to a child. "I was straight with you from the beginning, but you chose not to hear me."

"I hear you now," she said firmly, shifting the door, ready to close it on him so that he wouldn't see her shatter. "I hear you loud and clear."

"Thank fuck!" he exclaimed, slapping his palms to his thighs.

Grace blinked, hating the tear that escaped her eye when she did. She didn't recognize the man standing on her porch. The gentle, caring, patient man she'd fallen in love with was nowhere in the stranger before her.

She pressed her lips together. "I'm so sorry that all I did was care for you and try to help you see that you're so much more than drugs and bad memories." She swallowed. "But, I get it; that's all you've known and anything else, anything new, frightens you to death."

Max glared at her, his gaze like pinpricks on her skin.

She lifted her chin toward Carter's car. "So go. If I truly was a mistake, and you feel nothing for me at all, it'll be easy as pie for you to leave. Right?"

Max huffed, his eyes flashing. "Right," he spat. He lips twitched as though he had more to say, but he simply exhaled and waved a dismissive hand. "Seriously, I don't need this shit."

He spun on his heel, thumped down the porch steps, and strode toward Carter's car, nearly pulling the door from the chassis. He threw himself down into the passenger seat and slammed the door. Grace watched the car reverse and disappear down the driveway before she stepped back into the house and closed the door gently. She put her back to it, and slid down until she met the floor.

It was only then that she broke apart into a million pieces.

28

Max was quiet. He was too quiet and, frankly, it was scaring the shit out of Carter.

Since leaving Grace's place he'd been silent, his deep breaths and tremoring hands obvious signs of the fury coursing through him. Carter hadn't asked what or why. He'd watched him talk to Grace, heard the raised voices through the windows of the Lexus, the hurt and fear plain as day on the two of them.

Carter sighed. What the hell was Max thinking? Carter had seen it on Grace's face. She was head over heels and, whether Max admitted it or not, he was more than a little fond of her in return. It broke Carter's heart seeing his friend deny himself happiness because of his fear, because of his past, because of a woman he still had on a pedestal. But what choice did he have? He had to support Max. Carter always had and that would never change.

Seeing Max so animated through the car windshield, however, regardless of the cause, was strangely comforting. It'd been too long since Carter had seen him passionate about something that was neither alcoholic or came in a small, see-through plastic bag. Grace seemed to have woken a part of Max that Carter had worried was lost. It was just cruel irony that Lizzie would decide to write to Max now, right when he was beginning to warm to the idea of moving forward.

But shit was never easy.

Carter turned the key in the lock of the Tribeca loft apartment he shared with Kat and opened the door, standing to the side to let

Max through. Carter shut the door behind them, his eyes immediately finding Kat sitting at the breakfast bar, wedding invitations covering almost all of it, amid envelopes, ribbon, and fancy calligraphy pens that she had insisted on buying. She looked up and smiled widely.

"Peaches," he whispered before he walked toward her. He leaned over the breakfast bar, placing a soft kiss on her mouth.

"Hey." She smiled against his lips. She looked over to Max, who was shuffling on his spot by the sofa. "It's good to see you, Max," she said softly. "You look well."

"You, too."

Carter had called Kat when Max had made his decision to return to New York, the sound of her voice in his ear the antidote he needed for the worry gripping his insides. Seriously, if Max stumbled back into his drugs and drinking because of Lizzie and her bullshit, Carter knew he'd scour the earth looking for her and make her pay dearly. At Carter's insistence, Max had called Tate on the plane, not that he'd said much, but it eased a part of Carter knowing that his best friend had people ready to rally around should shit go south.

Carter smiled gently at Max. "You hungry? I could fix something."

Max frowned. "You? Cook?"

Kat snickered and looked down at the RSVP in her hand.

"Well, no," Carter answered while scratching his cheek. "But I know how to order a pizza."

Max's smile was small, but it was there. "No, man. I . . . I think I'll turn in, if that's okay?"

Carter's eyes drifted to the clock on the wall. It was a little after 9 p.m. "Sure."

"I put new sheets on the bed and there's a towel there if you want a shower," Kat offered.

Max dipped his chin a little. "Thanks."

He grabbed his bag from where Carter had placed it by the door and wandered through the apartment toward the spare room. Carter exhaled when he heard the door click shut.

"You okay?" Kat asked, pushing her hand into his and squeezing.

Carter shook his head. "I'm worried about him."

Kat stood from her seat and walked around the breakfast bar. She wrapped her arms around Carter's neck and held him tightly. "I know, sweetheart. I know."

. . . .

Max was still awake at 3 a.m.

He'd dozed on and off for a few hours, played on his phone, taken a pill, but nothing seemed to work. He scowled accusingly at the crumpled envelope he'd placed on the bedside table. Max must have read the letter at least twenty times and each time it caused his lungs to contract and his heart to pound. Parts of what was written flittered through his mind, tumbling and scratching at wounds he thought long ago healed.

> *Max, I've picked up this pen so many times over the years, thinking I was ready to write this letter . . . I'd really like to see you . . . If we could talk . . . I know you might not want to . . . What I did was inexcusable . . . There are things to say. I'll be in New York for a week . . .*

His mind reeled, never slowing down, or shutting the hell up long enough for him to fall into a deep sleep. It was relentless.

The last good night's sleep he'd had—fuck . . . he'd slept next to Grace.

With that thought, Max shoved the covers away in frustration, grabbed a pair of sleep pants from his bag, and snuck out of the bedroom into the apartment, his bare feet quiet on the wooden floor. Making his way into the apartment proper, where the kitchen was set off from the living room, Max stutter-stepped when he realized Kat was also awake, sitting at the breakfast bar where he and Carter had found her when they arrived, the small light from under the stove hood the only illumination. She looked up, seemingly unsurprised to see him there.

"Hey. Everything okay?" she asked before he could turn and run.

He crossed his arms over his bare chest. "Um . . . can't sleep."

"Me either." She looked back down at the book lying open on the bar. She turned a page. "Wedding plans are not conducive to a good night's sleep." She smirked. "Except if your name is Wesley Carter." Her eyes found the direction of their bedroom. "Man could sleep through World War Three."

Max smiled. "He always was a heavy sleeper."

Kat sighed. "Do you want a hot drink? I have cocoa. I was just debating whether or not to have one to help me sleep."

Max took another step closer, warmed by her sincerity. "Sure."

He watched Kat lift from her seat and start moving around the kitchen, grabbing milk, cocoa powder, and cups. He parked his ass on the seat opposite hers and glanced down at what she'd been reading. It was a wedding catalog.

"Carter tell you that I'm driving him crazy with all this?" She gestured with a wave of her hand toward a pile of dried flowers, ribbons, fabric samples, and other terrifying wedding-type horrors sitting on the kitchen counter.

"No," Max replied quickly.

Kat caught his eyes. "You're as bad a liar as he is."

Max snorted quietly. "He may have mentioned it. But he just wants you to be happy."

He saw a smile pull at the side of her mouth as she poured hot water into the cups. "I am." She brought the cups over, placing one in front of him. "See that drawer by your knees?"

Max looked down, noticing a hole in the wood of the breakfast bar big enough for the tip of an index finger. "Yeah."

"Open it, would you?"

Max did as she asked and grinned when he saw what was in it. Packs of Oreos, chocolate with Oreo pieces, and all manner of other cookie treats filled the drawer. He looked up at her with wide, amazed eyes. "This his secret stash?"

Kat shrugged, a mischievous glint in her eye. "He *thinks* it's secret. Just like the one in his man cave at the beach house."

Max pulled out a pack of Oreos. "Bastard would never give up where he kept them. It was always a nightmare when we partied here and got a mad case of the munchies."

He tore the pack open, taking one for himself, and offered them over to Kat. She took one and dipped it into her cocoa.

"How'd you get it out of him?"

Kat smiled into her cup. "I didn't. I have ninja-level stealth skills."

Max nodded, impressed. "Nice."

"I'm marrying him; I know everything there is to know."

Yeah, just like he and Lizzie had been. Max's smile faded. He sipped his cocoa as a feeling of panic and anxiety, the likes of which he'd not felt since before rehab, skittered across his neck.

"I'm sure it'll be all right," Kat said, her face open and honest, apparently seeing the stress he was trying so hard to hide. "Whatever you decide."

Max swallowed and rested his elbows on the breakfast bar between them. "Carter told you everything, huh?"

"Does that bother you?" Kat asked cautiously.

Max thought about it for a moment, but shook his head. "I'm glad he has you."

They sat then in comfortable silence, eating cookies and drinking cocoa, before Max said, "Do *you* think I'm an idiot?"

Kat's gaze snapped to his, surprise prevalent. "An idiot? I—I'm not sure—"

Max held a hand up, smiling. "It's okay. Honestly." He shrugged.

"I know we've never really . . . talked or anything, but I'd like to hear what you think. I know Carter thinks I'm crazy coming back." He laced his fingers around his cup, his shoulders sagging with the weight of the world. "*Am* I fuckin' stupid for even thinking of doing this?"

Kat sat back, as though carefully considering her answer. Her green eyes were intense on him and, for a split second, Grace's face flashed in Max's mind. He blinked slowly, waiting.

"I think . . ." Kat started. She glanced at her cup and gradually sat forward. "I think that you need to do what *you* feel is right."

Max exhaled in frustration and opened his mouth to tell Kat what a crock-of-shit answer that was. She held up her palm and cocked an eyebrow. "I haven't finished."

He could clearly see what Carter loved so much about her; she was sassy and Max was damn sure she put Carter in his place all the time.

"I also think that you're very brave," she added.

That brought Max up short. Brave? He didn't think so. He'd never felt more terrified. He shook his head gently.

"You're willing to face what nearly broke you," Kat murmured. "That's very brave."

Max clenched his teeth, holding back the angry retort that threatened; he had no right. He'd asked for her opinion. An opinion that itched like an insect bite. But how could he refute what Kat had said? Lizzie *had* nearly broken him. He'd fallen apart without her, because of her. If they met, would he shatter all over again? He'd grown so used to the sensation of being whole over the past few months, he wasn't sure he'd survive even the most gentle of taps from her.

"Has Carter ever told you about my grandmother, Nana Boo?" Kat asked.

Max nodded, not looking up. "Yeah, he's mentioned her. She's the one who makes him the killer Oreo cheesecake, right?"

Kat laughed. "She does. Every time she visits. I swear, he should be, like, three hundred pounds." Max chuckled despite himself. "She's the very best person I know. I still go to her about everything. When I was in senior year, I had my first boyfriend. I was eighteen and madly in love, while he was apparently madly in love with three other girls behind my back."

Max's eyes found hers. "Ouch."

Kat lifted her eyebrows. "Right? So we broke up. Three months later he called me up, begging for me to take him back, he was sorry, he wouldn't do it again, blah, blah, blah. I went to Nana Boo to ask what she thought I should do."

Max sat forward. "And what did she say?"

Kat swallowed her sip of cocoa. "She said, Katherine, angel, never answer the door when the past comes knocking." Her voice grew softer. "It never has anything new to say."

Max took a deep breath, the echo of her words reverberating through him. He slumped in his seat and stared at the breakfast bar suddenly feeling nothing but defeated. He was so fucking confused. His body torn in two. His mind wanting one thing—to walk away from what nearly killed him—and his heart wanting another. It was exhausting. The edges of his brain teased with a righteous headache and, for the first time in months, he craved a line.

Angry with himself, he pressed the heels of his hands to his eyes until he saw small white stars dancing behind his eyelids.

"Do me a favor, Max, will you?"

Kat's request brought Max's head up, blinking away the fuzzy darkness. "Sure."

"Be careful." Kat reached over, placed a small hand on his forearm, and squeezed. "You have a lot of people who care and who worry about you. Don't forget that, okay? You're not alone." She smiled gently. "We're family."

Max's throat grew impossibly tight. He nodded jerkily in reply.

Kat gave his arm one last squeeze and glanced at the clock. "Damn. I need to get to bed. Some of us have work tomorrow."

She smiled and lifted from her seat, collecting the cups and placing them in the sink while Max tucked the pack of Oreos back in Carter's not-so-secret drawer. He stood as Kat passed him.

"Hey, Kat?" She turned with a small smile. "Thanks."

She dipped her head. "Sure, Max. Any time."

.   .   .

Three days passed and, with each one, Max knew his window for meeting Lizzie was slowly closing; she was only in town for another four.

He'd kept himself busy, meeting Tate, having a session with Elliot, and attending a local NA meeting that Carter found on the Internet. Max could see the worry in the eyes of the people around him, the anticipation as they waited for him to make a final decision, and hoped that his proactive approach to his continuing recovery would ease their concerns a little. And they had every right to be concerned; the cold fingers of addiction had reemerged with a vengeance, whispering sweet nothings into Max's ear when he was alone, like the damn devil on his shoulder it was.

He hung out at the body shop, even helping Riley fix a sweet Ferrari 250 GT that just ached for his foot on her gas pedal. The smell of grease and metal and the thump of rock music were a welcome relief from the bullshit that had been flying around his head for days, and helped him realize how much he loved what he did. He went over paperwork, began organizing Carter's bachelor party, and ran.

He ran a lot. He ran through Central Park, he ran along the Hudson, he ran anywhere he could in an attempt to clear his mind. It was of little surprise that at those times, he thought about Grace the most. She'd been his running partner for months, so it was to be expected. At least that's what he told himself as his feet pounded the asphalt.

He hadn't heard from her since he'd left Preston County, and part of him, a very small part, was relieved. He'd resisted the urge to text or call, having no idea what he would say anyway. Truthfully, he was still stewing, still deliberating over what she'd said to him . . . but he tried his best not to dwell, not to think about her and what she was doing. He told himself frequently that he had no right. But still, his mind wandered back to her.

It was afternoon on the fourth day, while he was running, that Max at last made his decision.

After making a phone call to Carter's office, he headed downtown to WCS Communications, Carter's company, admiring the swanky décor of the lobby, thinking that maybe he should have changed out of his running gear beforehand, and rode the elevator up to the fortieth floor.

Carter's PA, Martha, smiled as he approached her desk. "Max?" Max nodded and Martha waved toward a door. "He's waiting for you."

He pushed the large wooden door open to find Carter standing at a window that boasted a hell of a view over the financial district. It was a gorgeous summer day in the city, and Max was somewhat relieved that he didn't suffer from vertigo. Shit looked a long way down from up here. Carter turned when he heard the door click shut; his face was nervous. He tried to smile past it, but, after twenty years of friendship, Max could see through that shit like crystal.

"You're going to see her," Carter said, as Max opened his mouth.

Apparently Max was just as transparent. He pushed his hands into the pockets of his running shorts. "I don't think I have another choice here, man."

Carter rubbed a palm over his chin. "You do, Max. You do. But I know you'll beat yourself up if you don't go."

Max lifted his shoulders. "I have to know," he confessed quietly. "I have to know . . . why."

"I know." Carter moved closer.

Max sensed his friend's disappointment, but he couldn't let that sway him. He'd made a decision and he would stick with it, for his own peace of mind.

"So what's the plan?" Carter asked, guiding Max toward a brown leather corner sofa. "How do you wanna do this?" He unfastened the single button on his navy blue suit jacket and sat down.

Max sat with him and pulled his cell out. "I'm gonna text her. I thought about calling but . . . I don't know what hearing her voice will do to me."

Carter was silent for so long, Max looked up from the phone in his hand. Carter sat back, his gaze on the carpet, pressing the backs of his fingers to his lips, looking for all the world as scared as Max felt. "You're sure?" he asked quietly.

Max nodded and pulled from his pocket the battered letter that held Lizzie's phone number. He took a deep breath and began typing. His text message was short and to the point: *I can meet you. Tomorrow. Max.*

Once done, his thumb hovered indecisively over the send button. He paused, his head suddenly echoing with Grace's words: *Tell me you didn't feel something last night. Tell me it meant nothing to you . . . ,* along with the image of her face as it collapsed when he'd fired back, so irate and stubborn.

He ground his teeth, hating how the memory made him feel, hating how what she'd asked him poked at parts of himself that scared Max to death, knowing what he'd said to her was unforgivable and categorically untrue. He growled deep in his chest and shook off the guilt.

He slapped the pad of his thumb down on the screen defiantly and pressed send.

Because fuck it, that's why.

He breathed through the thundering pulse in his ears while Carter sat stock-still at his side, seemingly without words. Both men stared at the phone, apprehension pulsing between them.

Lizzie's reply came within a minute: I'm staying at the Hilton in Midtown. One o'clock in the lobby?

That was no good. Familiar ground was important if this was going to work.

One o'clock. Sam's Diner across the street from the Hilton.

Okay. Thank you, Max.

Max pressed a button to quickly black out his cell phone screen and Lizzie's gratitude, and slumped back into the sofa, eyes closed, nausea rippling through him as though Lizzie's text was a big-ass stone thrown into his relatively peaceful little world. He couldn't figure it. Surely, he should have felt some sort of satisfaction, some sort of revelation with contacting her after so long.

But, no; all he felt was distracted. Pressure on his chest transported him back to their old apartment, to the day Lizzie left, Max on his knees, frantically calling everyone he knew in an effort to find her. The memories trickled through before the levees broke and they slammed into him, thick and fast, like white-tipped rapids, pulling him under, swirling him around, with no pause for him to catch his breath.

"You're okay," Carter murmured at his side. "Breathe."

Bizarrely, with Carter's words, an image of Grace dancing by the moonlit lake on Fourth of July weekend slipped between the chaos. Along with the echo of her laugh, her arms above her head as she twirled, and the memory of her skin under his fingers, Carter's hand on Max's shoulder was the only thing keeping his ass securely on the sofa and not bolting out the door to find the nearest dealer.

29

Max stood outside the diner the following day, wondering whether it was at all possible for his heart to break his ribs. It pounded so hard, it almost hurt, and every time he attempted to move forward, to enter the place, it stuttered and squeezed. He was bone tired, having not slept a wink the entire night, worrying and hypothesizing about what the hell Lizzie could have to say, what *he* would say.

Dragging his feet, he pushed the door open. The smell of coffee and pancakes accosted him immediately, causing his stomach to roil. He glanced around the place, sweat dripping down his neck. She hadn't arrived. Relieved that he had more time to collect himself, Max commandeered an empty booth and slid into it, fisting his hands together on the tabletop. A waitress approached with a wide smile and a name badge that read "Grace." Max blew out a disbelieving breath. Wasn't that just the last thing he needed to see?

"Fuck's sake," he mumbled into his hand before he swallowed and ordered a coffee, wishing to God it could arrive loaded with alcohol to help calm his nerves and extinguish the memory of Grace and the look of concentration on her face when she took her damned photographs, that same look that had been plaguing him since he'd awoken that morning.

He shifted in his seat. He needed to get a serious grip. Maybe he should have agreed when Carter offered to wait with him until Lizzie arrived. At this rate, he was going to fidget and vibrate his way into an early grave. He simply couldn't sit still. Grace the Waitress placed his coffee in front of him at the same time the bell above the diner door rang.

Without even looking up, Max knew it was Lizzie. His skin suddenly felt too tight, pressing on him, making him breathless.

He looked up slowly, catching her eye.

Jesus.

She was the woman he remembered, but somehow different.

She began to approach, steady but timid. Her blonde hair, which she'd always worn long, was now shaped into a sophisticated bob that hung just under her chin. Her face was the same, small and thin, but now bore lines that Max couldn't seem to recall her having before, while her blue eyes, which he'd adored, were less sparkly and more calm, more mature. He was more than a little comforted that the dead look he'd seen in them the last few months they were together was nowhere in sight.

Her gaze stayed on him until she stood at the side of the table. Max hadn't even had the wherewithal to stand. He sat back in his seat, looking up at her, not knowing what to do or say.

"Hi," she said softly, tucking her hair behind her ears.

That'd be a good start, he supposed.

Max cleared his throat. "Hi."

Her lips pulled into a tremulous smile. "May I sit?"

Max nodded. "Sure."

She dropped her red bag onto the seat opposite and slid in. Max took the time to watch her, trying to see the woman he'd cherished for so long. He wasn't sure whether he succeeded. She was still devastatingly striking; her white vest top showed off her unblemished skin and delicate collarbone, while her stone-washed, knee-ripped jeans he'd noticed as she came near highlighted how petite she still was.

It was a strange paradox being confronted with this part of his past. A part that had been, at one stage, all he knew, all he cared about, wanted, and loved, and yet, sitting there with Lizzie in front of him, the surreal unfamiliarity of it all settled on him like a lead weight.

Grace the Waitress appeared at their table again before either of them could speak. Lizzie looked at Max's cup.

"Coffee," he offered.

Lizzie dipped her chin, then addressed their server: "Same, please."

They sat as the other people in the diner milled around them, and stared at each other in a way that was neither affectionate nor uncomfortable. Lizzie fiddled with a ring on her index finger. Max noted that there wasn't one on her wedding-ring finger. He wondered fleetingly what had happened to the engagement ring he'd bought her.

"Thank you for coming," she said quietly toward her coffee once it arrived. "I wasn't sure you'd come."

"I wasn't sure, either," Max admitted, his voice gruff with nerves.

She tilted her head toward her shoulder and poured milk into her cup. "I wouldn't have blamed you if you hadn't." She settled the milk down and looked back at him, her gaze meandering over his face and chest. "You look well. Different, but well."

Max glanced down at himself, pondering what changes she saw. "You, too," he offered instead, hating how his voice caught on every word.

She blushed a little. He'd never seen her do that when they were together. She'd always been so confident, so strong and formidable. He wasn't sure he liked it, but he had to accept, considering what she'd been through, what they'd both been through, there were bound to be differences. They weren't the same people, and that filled Max with a profound sense of sadness.

"I'm glad you got my letter. I wasn't sure you'd still live in the city. Do you still have the shop?" Lizzie asked.

Max nodded. "Same shop, same apartment." He sipped his coffee, the awkwardness of small talk almost intolerable. "You?"

She shook her head. "I moved back to Florida for a while, stayed with my family. I'm working now and have a small place." She smiled. "I like it. I'm happy."

Max swallowed, not returning her smile. If nothing else, in spite of their history, all he'd ever wished for her were good things. "I'm glad it worked out for you."

Even though it was the absolute truth, annoyance slithered across his back. "So is that why I'm here, for you to gloat and tell me how happy you are?"

Despite his best efforts to stop it, his voice was clipped and bitter, but, to her credit, Lizzie didn't react other than to shake her head.

"No," she replied softly. "That's not why I wrote." She took a deep breath and paused. "I . . . wrote because, after everything that happened between us, after losing . . . him, I wanted the opportunity to explain."

"So explain," Max said unsympathetically.

Lizzie licked her lips. "After he died, I wasn't the person you met, the person you loved. I didn't like who I became." Her gaze drifted to Max's hands. "I was so lost. I was . . . broken."

Max inhaled through his nose, sitting back. "And I wasn't?"

"I know you were," she answered quietly. "That's why we couldn't help each other. That's why I had to leave."

As much as he wanted to understand and accept what she was saying, Max couldn't help but feel cheated. "Yeah, you left," he said toward his cup. "After everything that happened between us. You left me without a word, no letter, no note, no postcard when you got to wherever the fuck you went. Nothing." Although his temper had begun to rally, Max's voice remained calm and level.

"I know." Lizzie closed her eyes slowly, making Max's teeth grind. If she began to cry, he didn't know what he might do. Walking out seemed like the best response, but he wasn't sure he'd be able to. "You have no idea how hard it was for me to leave, Max. I swear. I wanted to get in touch, but . . . I was so scared and then it seemed like it was too late."

"And now?"

Lizzie sighed. "I knew I was going to be in New York. And I guess I got to the point where I had to see you again, to tell you why. It seemed like the perfect chance. I realized that, if I know you at all, you'd need that much." She ran a hand through her hair. "I wanted the opportunity to tell you how sorry I am."

And then she stared at him, blue eyes beautiful and blazing, as if she'd rehearsed what she was about to say a thousand times. "I'm so sorry, Max," she whispered. "I'm so sorry I lost him. I'm so sorry that I couldn't help you, help us through it, and that I left you alone when I knew it would devastate you. I'm just so sorry for everything, and I know I don't deserve it, but I hope you can find it in yourself to someday forgive me."

Max opened his mouth to respond, but no words came, blocked by the sudden shock of emotion swelling in his throat. Lizzie became blurry as tears filled his eyes. He looked toward the windows of the diner, angry and willing them away, breathing through pursed lips. "You nearly killed me," he uttered, staring at the ceiling for a moment before turning back to her. "Do you understand that? You nearly *killed* me." He shook his head. "To lose Christopher was one thing, but to then lose you— I . . . Jesus, Lizzie, it was like I died."

Tears slipped down her cheeks then, but Max didn't care. It was more emotion than he ever remembered seeing from her after they lost their son and, in a strange way, it was comforting. It meant that she was alive again inside, aware, and breathing.

"You said his name," she croaked, smiling through her tears.

Max frowned. "Of course. He was my son."

"You were never able to say it. It's good to hear."

Max sniffed. "I guess therapy and rehab has its uses."

Lizzie's eyes widened. She nodded slowly. "Therapy helped me." She laughed humorlessly. "Although I still struggle with his name, I wouldn't be sitting here without it."

Max's temper slowly cooled while he watched her wipe the tears from her face with a napkin. "Did you think of me at all?"

The words slipped from his mouth before he could stop them.

Lizzie looked up, seemingly surprised by his question. "Every day," she replied softly. Max nodded shortly. "And you?"

"Yes," he said, looking down at the table. "I hated you for it."

"I understand." She sat back, not appearing hurt. "How are you, Max, really?"

He shrugged, wanting to be honest. "I'm . . . okay. Surviving. Living from one day to the next."

"And you have someone, someone who makes you happy?"

Grace's laughing face immediately flashed through Max's mind, stealing his breath away. "I—I'm not . . ." He shook his head. "It's not . . ."

Lizzie smiled. "It's all right." She rubbed her hands on her thighs. "I've been seeing someone for a couple of months. Nothing serious. But . . . it's nice. I like that I want to date again."

Max prepared himself for the devastating impact those words would bring, but, oddly, the pain never came. How could that be? He'd loved this woman, spent years with her, worshipped her body, breathed every inch of her in, and yet the indifference that settled over him, knowing that she was seeing someone else, was like a warm blanket, easing the pressure that had built in his chest since the day her letter had arrived.

They sat for the next hour, talking. It was stilted and awkward, like a couple on a first date. They shared their experiences of therapy, how their recoveries were going, and how old friends were. She asked about Carter and he asked about her family; she told him about moving into her new place and he told her about Preston

County, leaving out certain details though they drifted through his mind like leaves on a breeze. She apologized repeatedly and, despite the sincerity with which she offered her remorse, Max felt neither comforted nor fulfilled by it, as though her repentance made no difference to the past or the present he now lived.

"So, I have something for you," Lizzie said, pulling her bag closer and delving into it. She rummaged through it, frowning. "Dammit. I must have left them."

"What?"

"They're in my room at the hotel," she grumbled. "I was so stressed about today, I . . . would you mind if I went to get them?"

"What is it?"

She suddenly looked embarrassed. "It's just something that I need you to have."

Max cocked an intrigued eyebrow. "Okay."

She paused for a moment, regarding him carefully. "Why don't you come with me? I won't be long."

In her room? Max was shaking his head before he was speaking. "I don't think that's—"

Lizzie's laugh was loud and unexpected. "Really? What do you think will happen?"

Actually, Max wasn't sure, but being alone with her in a hotel room didn't make him feel as comfortable as it probably should have. He licked his lips.

"Fine," he said, realizing how ridiculous he sounded. "I should be heading back anyway."

She stood from her seat. Max threw money onto the table and followed Lizzie through the diner, out of the door, across the street, and into the lobby of the Hilton hotel.

. . . .

The elevator ride to her room was quiet except for the small ding punctuating each floor they ascended. Max caught Lizzie's reflection in the smooth steel of the door, noticing how much calmer she looked from when she first came into the diner. The lines on her face had all but disappeared and she stood taller, straighter, as though their conversation had lifted something from her. If he were honest, Max felt the same way. He felt less burdened, less heavy with the past.

The elevator reached floor twenty and Max followed Lizzie out of it and down the hall to her room. She unlocked the door and gestured for him to enter. He did as she asked, catching a breath of her perfume, sweet and unfamiliar. Standing with his hands in his jeans pockets, Max glanced from Lizzie, who closed the door, to the window, to the bed, and back again. His pulse picked up as panic began to take hold.

What the hell was he doing?

"Here."

Lizzie's voice came from his side. He looked down to see her holding a large bundle of envelopes, tied together with a blue ribbon. He took them cautiously, noting his name and address on the top one.

"What's this?"

"I wrote you a letter every day I was in therapy. It was part of my recovery," she murmured, her stare on the envelopes. "Each one tells you what I was going through, how I felt about you, how I felt about losing . . . Christopher."

Max's breath faltered as he held them tightly, overwhelmed and sad. "I don't know what to say," he confessed, meeting her gaze.

"You don't have to say anything," she replied. "I want you to have them. I want to explain and they say what I can't right now."

He turned them over in his hand and nodded. "Okay." He stood staring at them before he glanced toward the door. "Look, I'd better go."

She nodded and gradually moved to the side, allowing him to pass. "Max?"

He turned and, for a split moment, he saw the girl he remembered, lovely and ready to take life by the balls. "Yeah?"

"Could we . . . I mean, you have my number, can I— I'd like to stay in touch, maybe see you again."

Max blew out a confused breath. "I don't know, Liz. I mean"— he opened his arms, gesturing toward her and the room—"it's . . . this is all—"

"Overwhelming."

He dropped his arms to his sides. "Yeah."

She dipped her chin. "I get it."

Max stared at her, knowing her well enough to see that she had more to say. He waited.

"Can we . . ." She shifted where she stood. "I'd like it if we could hug it out."

She looked so earnest, so hopeful, that Max nodded before he could think clearly about it. Steadily, she drew closer and lifted her arms, sliding them around his neck, and pulled him close. Max's hands moved around her waist, returning the hug carefully. It was only when Lizzie lifted her nose to his neck and tightened her grip on him that he gave himself over to it, closing his eyes and resting his cheek against hers, understanding that it was a hug of apology for both of them, a hug of forgiveness, a hug that quietly and respectfully acknowledged the harrowing journey they'd shared.

"Thank you," she mumbled into his skin. "Thank you for today."

Max nodded, feeling her fingers play in the hair at his neck just as she used to do.

She hummed. "You smell the same."

Her words stirred something that felt like regret inside him. She didn't smell the same, she didn't smell of anything he recognized or wanted. Everything was so different. With a deep breath, he lifted his head but didn't loosen his hold. "Lizzie?" She opened her eyes. "I have to go."

"I know." She bit her lip, her gaze turning wary. "But I'm afraid to let go again."

More than a little surprised by her confession, Max stared at her for the length of three heartbeats. She stared back, took a deep, unwavering breath, then kissed him.

It lingered at the side of his mouth, tender and soft. Without thought, Max turned his head into it, capturing her gasp when he responded. Years ago that sound would have had Max desperate to have her, against the wall if necessary, but right then the sound caused his stomach to tilt as though he were at the top of a roller-coaster track and about to plummet to the ground. The kiss unbalanced him, made him dizzy, as if his body couldn't quite accept what was happening.

He didn't understand. Lizzie's lips *should* have been familiar—he'd kissed them a million times before—but now they felt strange, alien, and didn't taste the way he wanted them to, and her scent wasn't cocoa butter but different and, God fucking dammit, why the hell was he thinking about Grace when Lizzie was kissing him?

Wasn't this what he wanted? Wasn't this what he'd hoped for? Didn't he want the chance of being with Lizzie again after everything that had been before?

"No," he mumbled against her mouth, answering his unspoken question aloud.

He didn't. It wasn't right. Not now. They were different people, wanting different things. There wasn't even a glimmer of sweet nostalgia, of happier moments, when they would feast on each other for hours. Her kiss simply reminded him of a time in his life that he would never forget but was ready to move forward from.

He gripped Lizzie's waist. "No," he repeated. He pushed her away gently, spotting the high flush in her cheeks and the lust in her eyes.

"Oh God, Max," she exclaimed, hiding her mouth with her palm and stepping back. "I'm so sorry. I shouldn't have—I never should have . . . I don't know what I was thinking."

Max closed his eyes, her protests reminding him of the way Grace had apologized for kissing him, her mumblings, her shock, and the taste of her on his tongue when he'd reciprocated with more passion than he'd ever felt in his life.

Standing there staring at Lizzie, with the odd sensation of her mouth still tingling across his lips, as God was his witness, Max would have given anything for it to have been Grace instead. He'd have given anything to get the chance to kiss her again, to kiss her the way she deserved, to push into her body and hear her call out for him, to hold her and make her laugh.

He coughed, almost choking on those realizations as they flooded through him, sweeping away all the panic and anxiety of the last week, leaving nothing but hope and determination and something that felt suspiciously like love in their wake.

Looking down at himself, as though just realizing where he was, he blurted, "I have to go."

Lizzie crossed her arms over her chest. "Okay."

Max ran his hand through his hair, his heart pounding furiously with the need to get away, to get back to Preston County, back to Grace. He looked down at the envelopes still in his grasp, knowing that, as easy as it would have been to get the answers he'd thought he needed, they were too late. Silently, he placed them on a table located at the side of the hotel room door.

"I'll leave these here," Max said gently as he pulled out the most recent letter from the back pocket of his jeans and laid it on the top of the rest.

"Are you sure?" Lizzie asked, although her expression changed imperceptibly into one of understanding.

"Yeah," Max answered with a small smile. "I think we've said all there is to say."

The left side of Lizzie's mouth lifted in agreement. "She's a lucky girl, Max."

Max startled.

"Whoever it is that you're going back to. I'm glad you learned to love again," she admitted. "You deserve it."

Her words squeezed a cold, dark piece of him, resuscitating it, while simultaneously blowing the cobwebs off all the other parts he thought lifeless, the parts he knew wanted Grace, needed Grace, suddenly missed Grace more than he would ever be able to explain.

Max stepped forward and placed a small kiss on Lizzie's cheek. "Take care, yeah?" he whispered.

"I will. You, too."

Without another word, Max turned and walked out of the room. The sound of the door shutting behind him echoed down the long corridor like a welcome death knell to all the bullshit that had made Max who he was. He knew that, by walking away, he could finally let go of his past and begin to start living again, and as the distance between he and Lizzie grew, he became more and more determined to have Grace at his side every step of the way.

30

Max slammed Carter's apartment door shut, cell phone in his hand, cursing the fucking thing up and down. He was so involved in his argument with the inanimate piece of shit that he didn't notice Carter and Riley, standing, looking surprised, as though they'd shot up from their seats on the sofa. Max came to an abrupt halt when he saw them both and glanced around the apartment in confusion. "I thought you went to work?"

"I went in," Carter explained, "and then took the rest of the day off in case you needed me. And Riley dropped by—"

"Because he was freaking out," Riley interrupted. "And clucking like a mother hen."

"I wasn't freaking," Carter argued, shooting Riley a narrowed glare. "I was just worried." Carter looked back over at Max, his expression suggesting he expected to see Max covered in blood and other battle wounds. "So what happened? How did it go?"

Max blinked and took a deep breath, staring down at his phone. "I have to get a hold of Grace."

Carter's face creased in puzzlement. "Grace?"

"Grace?" Riley echoed. "Oh! Running girl. Your fuck buddy."

Carter elbowed Riley. "Dude!" He turned back to Max. "Why do you need to get a hold of Grace? What about Lizzie? What do you—?"

"Grace!" Max said loudly, waving his cell as though that would explain everything. "I've called her but her phone's turned off, or she's blocked me, which is absolutely possible, and I wouldn't blame her. I've called Whiskey's but Holly won't tell me anything and Uncle Vince said she left Preston County the day after me, saying something about her photographs. I don't know where she would have gone other than DC, but what the fuck am I supposed to do—"

"Max!"

Max's mouth shut as the sound of his name rattled around the apartment. Expecting to see Carter looking annoyed, he was surprised as hell to see a wide smile pulling at his friend's face. Max stepped back nervously. "What?"

"You want to speak to Grace?" Carter asked, cocking his head to the side. "You need to see her?"

"Yeah." Max ran a hand through his hair. "Seeing Lizzie and realizing that I . . . I have to talk to Grace—I just want to explain that I . . . to tell her that—you know, that . . ."

Carter's smile grew softer. "That you love her."

Max's eyes snapped to Carter's, then to Riley's, and back again, narrowing quickly. He pointed an accusatory finger at the pair of them. "You fuckin' knew!"

Riley snickered and Carter barked a laugh. "Of course we fuckin' knew. I knew the minute I saw the two of you at the damned boardinghouse all puppy-eyed and shit."

"And it was pretty obvious the day Tate and I visited," Riley chimed in, looking pleased as shit.

"And why the fuck didn't you tell me?" Max asked in disbelief.

Carter crossed his arms over his chest. "Would it have made a difference?"

"Of course!"

Carter cocked an eyebrow and Riley snorted. All three men knew that answer was utter bullshit.

Max shifted his weight from one foot to the other. "I mean . . . maybe."

Carter took a step closer. "You said it yourself. You needed to see Lizzie. I know you, brother. You'll never be swayed or bullied into anything and you had to come to this realization yourself."

Max rubbed his eyes with the pads of his fingers, shuffled to the nearest chair, and dropped into it. "Realization," he mumbled, dropping his head back and glaring at the ceiling. "Is that what this is?"

Carter and Riley sat down on the sofa opposite. "You tell me," Carter uttered. "Do you love her?"

Max swallowed. Whatever was whirling through him damn sure felt like it. "I think so," he said quietly.

It was strange, though. When he'd fallen in love with Lizzie, it was like being hit across the head with a sledgehammer; he'd known it from minute one. This feeling with Grace, however, was more subtle, less obtrusive, less flash-bang, and more like a gentle tingle that covered his entire body and warmed him from the inside out, as though, over time, she'd snuck quietly, carefully, and planted herself into all the dark, barren parts that Max hid for fear of being hurt all over again. It was an altogether satisfying feeling that, until that moment, Max hadn't realized he'd wanted.

"I . . . I miss her," he admitted. "Shit, I can't stop thinking about her and when Lizzie kissed me all I thought about was Grace and how I wanted it to be her."

"What the fuck?" Riley exclaimed at the same time Carter shouted, "Lizzie *kissed* you?"

Max groaned, flailing and lifting his arms to the heavens. "Focus, guys. Jesus!"

Carter held his hands up in an effort to calm himself and Riley, who suddenly looked murderous. "Fine. Fine," Carter said, rubbing his hands across his head.

Max sat forward, his hands dropping between his knees. "I just . . . the thing that keeps coming back to me is, what can I really offer her?" He looked up at his friends. "I mean, how do I know if I can even give her what she wants? If I'm *still* what she wants." He thought back to the horrible things he'd said to her the day he left and cupped his hands to his face. "Fuck."

Carter sat back and cleared his throat. "Tell me somethin', when you were together, doin' your thing, did she ever say how she felt or tell you what she wanted?"

Max smiled toward the floor and nodded. "She said all she wanted to do was love me."

Riley shrugged. "Then let her. That's a gift right there, man."

"I want to," Max agreed. "I do."

Carter shifted again, moving closer to the edge of the couch. "I know you think you've nothing to offer anyone, Max, but trust me, you do. If this year has proved anything, it's that you're a strong son of a bitch who can get through just about anything."

Max's chest warmed. "But a relationship?"

Carter lifted a shoulder. "Why does it have to be called that? No labels, huh? Just talk to her and see what you both feel. Take it a step at a time."

Max's stare drifted back to his cell. "I have to find her first."

He sat back dejectedly at the same time Riley stood. "Then what the fuck are you still sitting there for?" he asked before slapping Max on the shoulder. "Let's go get your running girl."

That afternoon, Max, Riley, and Carter scoured the phone book and the Internet, trying to track down Grace's brother's club. It was the only lead Max had. It took nearly two hours of searching, the name Kai and DC being the only things they had to go on. Once they had four possible addresses, the three of them piled into Riley's Jeep and headed out. Max had to admit, the whole thing was kind of exciting. The thought of seeing Grace again was as terrifying as it was exhilarating, and Max spent the majority of the car ride going over in his mind just what he intended to say to her.

The first club they arrived at was boarded up, and had been for a while from the looks of the graffiti sprayed across the brickwork. Determined, they reached the second club by the early evening.

Kai's name on the owner plate was clear above the door of the place, filling Max with a ball of nervous energy so large he all but barged his way in. Nevertheless, all they found was a sassy woman with an incredible Afro and bright red lips behind the bar who, once she'd divulged that Kai was in New York, and upon hearing who it was they were also looking for, told them they had to leave before she had them thrown out by security. That was pretty much all the confirmation Max needed to realize that the woman knew Grace, but what more could he do? Even Riley couldn't seem to coax anything from her despite his wide smile and charm.

Undeterred, Max left his cell number and a note to Grace asking her to call along with the silent hope that the woman would pass it on, and tried like hell not to let Carter and Riley see the disappointment that tensed his shoulders and squeezed his heart.

That had been more than two weeks ago and Max was still no closer to finding Grace. His cell phone stayed infuriatingly quiet. Even though he'd asked his family and friends in Preston County to keep him up to date should Grace return, he'd slowly started to resign himself to the fact that he might never see her again, and that filled him with a profound hopelessness.

To divert his attention away from the hollow ache that had taken up residency in his chest, Max threw himself back into work, arriving at the shop bright and early every day and staying until late at night. He also decided to move back into his own apartment. He knew Carter stressed about Max being on his own, but truthfully, he needed the space to think and, with the wedding mere weeks away, he knew Carter and Kat didn't need him under their feet. He attended his meetings and continued his running, all the while wondering what Grace was doing, who she was with, and whether she thought of him at all.

The only silver lining amid the bullshit was that, since he'd said good-bye to Lizzie, the urge to go out and get high and shitfaced had lessened, changing from an all-out shout to a mere whisper. Max knew he'd done enough damage to let everyone down again with a damn relapse, and when he wasn't working, running, or attending meetings, Max would recall, unashamedly, the disappointment on Grace's face when he'd gotten drunk that night at the bar. Right or wrong, that shit always took the potency right out of his cravings.

It was after a long, hard day at the shop and Max was lounging on his sofa, eating pizza, and watching a shitty horror movie when there was a knock on the door. Curious and not expecting anyone, Max threw the pizza crust into the box and padded through his apartment.

He peered through the peephole and quickly opened the door. "Hey, man. You okay?"

Riley smiled. "Yeah, I'm good."

"Come in." Max stepped to the side, allowing him to enter. As pleasant a surprise as it was to see Riley, it was also unusual. Ordinarily, he would announce his impending arrival with either a phone call or a text. Max had received neither. "Can I get you something? I don't have alcohol, obviously, but I have juice, water, coffee."

Riley shook his head. "No, brother, I'm fine. I won't stay long."

Max frowned. "Sounds ominous."

Riley smiled again but this time it fell quickly. He pushed his hands into his pockets while his gaze wandered from the floor to a spot over Max's shoulder and back again.

Max took a step closer. "How was your day off? You all right?"

"I um . . . I have something for you, but I wanted to say a couple of things first."

Max nodded slowly. "Okay. Shoot."

Riley exhaled heavily. "I know what it's like," he murmured toward his shoes.

"You know what what's like, man?"

Riley's hazel stare found Max. "I know what it's like to lose the woman you love."

Thinking he was joking, the beginning of a laugh and an inappropriate comment pulled at Max's mouth, but it quickly fizzled out in his throat. From the expression on Riley's face, he was deadly serious.

"What? Love? How—you . . . *you?*" Max wasn't trying to be purposefully obtuse or mean, but Riley, in the almost ten years of their friendship, had never mentioned loving anything other than cars and one-night stands.

Riley breathed a despondent laugh. "Yeah, me." He rubbed a hand across his trimmed beard and sighed. "It's a long story, one that very few people know about, but . . . yeah." He shrugged. "I know people think I'm just some knuckleheaded womanizer who doesn't give a shit, and it's partly true, but there was a time when I wasn't, when I did give a shit about . . . someone."

Max shook his head. Seeing his friend so solemn, so uncharacteristically serious was more than a little unnerving. "Why . . . how did we not— Why didn't you say something?"

Riley gave a wry smile. "And shatter the illusion?" He cleared his throat. "Besides, I've no one to blame but myself." He furrowed his brow. "And it's ancient history."

Max wasn't entirely sure that was the truth, but he nodded to appease him.

"To get a second chance like this doesn't happen for many, Max."

"I know."

"A guy dropped by the shop yesterday while you were at your meeting with Elliot," Riley continued. "Dropped off a sweet '67 Mustang for an oil change. We got to talkin'. Turns out he owns some gallery space uptown. It's kind of a hobby of his, you know, helping young talent in the area to get noticed." He reached into his back pocket and pulled out a crumpled flyer. "He invited me to a photography and art show he's hosting there this weekend and, well, let's face it, Carter's ugly ass doesn't look as good in a suit as you do. So I wondered if you'd be my date."

He handed the flyer to Max, who was, despite his confusion, chuckling. He took the flyer sensing that he was missing something. He looked down at it and his mouth dropped open. "Holy shit."

"Yeah. I thought that's what you'd say."

Max's eyes traced Grace's name across the top of the flyer, alongside a photograph that he recognized from her living room in West Virginia. "Her show," he whispered. "Dammit, she took all those photos for this show she said she was doing and—I forgot . . . I didn't even know it was in New York."

"She'll be there," Riley said cautiously. "This might be the shot you've been waiting for."

Max stuttered. "I . . . I'm not sure if— Should I?" He wasn't certain arriving unexpectedly on Grace's big night was the right thing to do. He had no idea how she'd react.

Riley reached out and squeezed Max's shoulder. "I'll let you decide that." He patted him and maneuvered around Max to get back to the door. "Let me know what you want to do, okay?"

Max nodded, still staring at the flyer in his hand. "I will." He looked up. "Hey, Riley. Thanks, man."

Riley nodded. "Sure."

• • •

"Are you going?" Tate asked before he took a sip of the mango juice Max had poured for him.

"Of course," Max replied, sitting down in his usual chair while Tate all but lounged on the sofa. His T-shirt was faded black across which, in a familiar yellow font, it read, "Jedi on the streets. Sith in the sheets."

Max blinked in bewilderment before asking, "You don't think I should?"

Tate shook his head. "I'm with Elliot, I absolutely think you should go, but I'm wondering what you think will happen."

Max blew a breath between his lips, turning it into a raspberry. "Who knows? All I can do is hope she'll give me a chance and listen."

"And if she doesn't?"

"I wouldn't blame her. I was . . ."

"A fucking asshole."

"Yeah." Max snorted.

"But are you a fucking asshole who's going to hit something hard to ease the pain if she turns you down?" The serious concern in Tate's voice was punctuated by the way he stared at Max, who shifted uncomfortably in his seat. "Sorry. But I have to ask, buddy."

Max licked his lips. "Honestly? I haven't thought about drink or powder since I saw Lizzie." He glanced toward the living room window of his apartment and to the clear blue sky beyond it. "It's like, now that she and I have said good-bye, I can breathe. Like I got closure or something."

Tate's mouth pulled into a knowing smile. "Yeah, man. I hear ya."

The two men sat in silence for a moment before Max sat forward, lowering his voice despite the fact that they were alone. "So, will you tell me something about Riley?"

Tate blinked slowly. "If it's anything to do with Seb and me putting red juice powder mix in the showerhead before he used it, then I know nothing."

Max knew Seb to be the youngest of the Moore brothers. "Red juice mix?"

"Powder mixed with the water when he turned on the shower." Tate snickered. "Bathroom looked like that scene in *Carrie*. Mom nearly shit bricks; he scrubbed himself for damn near a week to get clean. Man, it was awesome."

Max rubbed his eyes with the pads of his fingers, tittering. "No, that wasn't it, but thanks for that visual. I was wondering if you knew who it was that he lost." Tate appeared perplexed. "A woman," Max clarified. "When he came over last night, he said something about knowing what it was like to lose the woman he loved."

It wasn't that Max was prying. Since Riley's visit, he'd been genuinely worried about the man and concerned that he'd known nothing about Riley's past and the obvious pain he'd suffered.

Tate took a deep breath and sat back gradually, all hints of joking and pranks forgotten. He rested his ankle on the opposite knee. "Yeah, I know who it was." Max waited, but Tate didn't embellish. His expression was firm. "It ain't my story to tell, man."

"I get it," Max offered, knowing a big brother's protectiveness and loyalty was not something to fuck with. "He's okay, though, right?"

Tate nodded. "I think so." He smirked. "Riley's like a bouncy ball, doesn't matter how hard you throw him, he always comes back harder and faster."

· · ·

At seven o'clock Saturday evening, decked out in black dress pants, white shirt, and a thin black tie he'd borrowed from Carter, Max sat in the passenger seat of Riley's Jeep as Riley drove the two of them across the city toward the art exhibition.

"You okay?" Riley asked for the fourth time since they'd left Max's place.

"Other than being dressed up fancier than I would be for a damn court appearance, I'm fine," Max answered with a sly grin.

"Prick," Riley muttered, shaking his head and fidgeting with his own tie. "The flyer said to dress sharp, so, shit, we dressed sharp." He glanced at himself in the rearview. "Damn sharp, baby, I look fucking hot."

Max chuckled and shook his head, his heart rate rising as they drew closer to Greenwich Village. He ran a hand down his tie and breathed deeply.

"You look okay, I guess," Riley muttered before grinning. "And you know, if this shit doesn't work out, we could always hit a couple of gay bars. We're in the area. You'd fit right in."

Rolling his eyes, Max shrugged. "I take that as a compliment."

"You should," Riley agreed seriously. "I'd do you."

Max laughed, knowing that Riley's incessant ramblings were an attempt to calm them both. Riley hadn't stopped twitching for the entire car journey. Max was honestly relieved that Carter hadn't joined them. He wasn't sure he would have been able to cope with the two of them fussing around him. Max wasn't naïve, of course; he knew having friends who cared about him was a great problem to have, especially when he considered the shit he'd put them all through. But Christ.

He turned to Riley. "Thanks for doing this."

Riley dipped his chin. "Any time, brother. You know that."

Riley parked the Jeep and the two of them sat for a minute, listening to the engine tick as it cooled. Max went over his well-thought-out spiel silently, swallowed down his fear, and climbed out onto the quiet, humid street. With Riley at his side, Max felt somewhat comforted. He damn sure knew he couldn't have done it alone.

The building they approached was fairly innocuous, save for the twelve-foot window affording a view inside it and an awesome banner that reached across the entire front declaring the show open and the names of the four artists, Grace's included, whose work was being shown. A guy at the door with a clipboard and a mustache that would have put Salvador Dalí to shame smiled as they drew near. Riley gave them his name and then a name Max had never heard of, presumably that of the owner Riley had met at the body shop.

"Ah, special guests," Dalí exclaimed with an extravagant wave of his hand. "Of course, of course, my darlings, go in. Enjoy!"

The two of them smiled nervously and, with Max in front,

slipped around him into the air-conditioned lobby. "What the fuck did you just do?" Max asked with a snicker.

"I have no idea," Riley answered, glancing back at the door, looking as though he was ready to beat a hasty retreat. "But I think he just slapped my ass."

Max laughed into his hand and shoved Riley toward a collection of paintings titled *Bask in Death*. Practically giggling like schoolchildren, the two of them came to an abrupt halt, eyeing the dark splashes of color against the whitewash of the gallery walls skeptically.

"Talk about a joy killer," Riley uttered while simultaneously grabbing two glasses of orange juice from a passing waiter.

Max nodded, not voicing his views about the work even though he quite liked them, and glanced around discreetly. He couldn't spot Grace amid the crowd of about one hundred people, and the anticipation built ever higher. He figured he may as well try to relax while he had the chance. He sipped the juice and meandered around the paintings, stopping at a couple and quietly losing himself in the colors, themes, and messages of each one. He'd never been one to really stop and appreciate art, despite his affinity for painting, and soon found himself enjoying it. Riley, meanwhile, tilted his head this way and that, trying to make heads or tails of the numerous canvases they passed, much to Max's amusement.

"I don't get it," Riley grumbled, after staring hard at a canvas that was bare but for a single orange circle in its center.

Max cocked an eyebrow, equally puzzled. "Yeah, I'm with you on that."

"Now these I like," Riley said, disappearing around a corner.

Max followed to find him standing in front of a wall covered in photographs. Some were small, no bigger than the size of a postcard, while others were at least three feet wide. Max immediately recognized the forests, the mountains, and the rocks that resided by a small cottage back in Preston County. Max looked at the title plaque. *Mind, Body, and Soul* by Grace Brooks. He smiled before he even felt the desire to do so; at the same time a swell of pride gathered in his chest.

"These are hers," he whispered.

The colors were extraordinary. Grace's eye for textures and light was glaringly obvious in each shot. The angles were precise and thought out, leaving the viewer disoriented in some and calm in others. This was definitely the mind part of her work. She'd had that effect on Max from the moment they met, all baffled and off kilter.

"They're great," Riley said after a quiet moment, gradually making his way around the next corner of the exhibit, where the lighting, Max noticed, was duller, and less like the harsh, bright white of the rest of the place.

Above this particular collection of photographs, painted directly onto the wall of the gallery in black cursive lettering, were the words "Hope for the Soul." The swelling in Max's chest receded as his gaze wandered over the black-and-white images littering the wall, replaced with the crushing weight of his guilt.

"Oh, Jesus," he mumbled, crossing one hand and arm over his stomach while cupping his mouth with the other.

"What?" Riley asked, looking up from one shot that Max remembered Grace taking as clearly as if it were yesterday.

"It's me," he croaked.

Riley frowned. "Are you serious?"

Max nodded and moved closer to the wall. The shots were taken the day he'd met her at the cottage, the day they'd sat on the overturned log and he'd touched her for the first time, his hands on her thighs. There were pictures of Max's face, arms, hands, but, to anyone else, including Riley, it was just some random man. Grace was right. No one would know it was Max but the two of them. Astounded, Max looked at every one, noticing some he didn't remember her taking, some that, from the wrinkles next to his eyes, he could tell he was laughing. In the few shots that showed his eyes, Max noticed, even in black-and-white, how happy he looked, how young and relaxed and, dare he say it, in love.

"I'm such a fucking fool," he murmured.

Riley smiled sympathetically before his gaze drifted from Max to something over Max's shoulder. "Dude."

Max stilled, knowing from Riley's expression who it was he'd seen. "Is it her?"

"Well, I've never seen her," Riley replied, moving closer to Max. "But I remember Tate's description just fine."

"Fuck," Max gasped as his pulse began to race.

Riley placed his hand on Max's shoulder in silent encouragement. "Be prepared, man," he said softly. "She looks fucking amazing."

With that comment, Max turned his head and looked over his shoulder. Sure enough, there was Grace and, sweet Jesus, Riley was right. Her hair was fastened in a tight bun at the top of her head, leaving soft curls that appeared crafted to the side of her face. With her hair up, her neck looked impossibly long, wrapped in a stunning necklace that glinted and sparkled under the bright gallery spotlights. Her dress was . . . *unbelievable*. It was a canary-yellow strapless number that reached the floor and pulled in at her waist, accentuating all of her glorious curves and the exquisite warm tones of her skin.

She was a vision and Max could barely breathe.

"You wanna go over?" Riley asked.

"Yeah, stay here," Max answered unthinkingly, turning around and taking the first of the fifteen wobbling steps it took to reach her, leaving Riley where he stood. As he drew closer, Max's stare stayed on Grace's shoulder blades, watching the way they moved as she talked with her hands, as she always did, recalling the way they felt under his hands and against his mouth as he moved in her.

He approached silently and stood a couple of feet behind Grace while she finished her conversation. The woman she was speaking to glanced alluringly over Grace's shoulder in Max's direction, alerting Grace to his presence. She turned to him, smile in full effect before she realized who he was. The smile fell like a stone in water, taking all of Max's courage and hope with it. Her green eyes flashed first with shock and then something Max couldn't quite identify. Nevertheless, it made him feel minute.

"What are you doing here?" she asked, her voice a staggered breath.

Max cleared his throat and cracked his knuckles. "I came to see you."

He glanced at the woman and her male companion pointedly. They mumbled their good-byes and moved toward another part of the gallery.

Grace watched them go before turning back to Max, bewilderment clear on her face. "How are— What? Why?"

Max coughed a nervous laugh. "Why?" he echoed, his spiel all but dissolving the longer he stood looking at her. "Well, I wanted to see if you were okay, and . . . I, um, I thought that we could talk. Maybe. If you wanted."

Grace stared at him as though he'd spoken in an alien language. "Talk," she repeated. "About what?" She licked her lips, her green eyes sad as she lifted her shoulders. "What is there left to say?"

"There's a lot left to say," Max replied, swallowing hard. "Things I need to say, want to say." He sighed. "I tried to find you."

She nodded toward her feet. "I know. Sienna told me you were at the club. I got your note. I thought about calling but . . ."

She looked at him, her honest gaze like a warm blanket over his entire body.

Christ, he'd missed her.

"But I can't do this right now, Max," she whispered.

Max took a step closer when she turned to go. "Gracie," he pleaded.

Her face pinched. "Please don't call me that."

The hurt in her words and the anguish tensing her shoulders was like a punch to the gut. "I'm sorry," Max blurted. "I'm sorry. I just wanted to ask you a question—what I said to you that day . . ."

"Hurt me more than—"

"I know."

"I never asked you for anything other than to let me in."

"I know. I've—I'll never—"

"Everything okay here, Grace?"

The man who approached was tall, strong, and sickeningly handsome. Max's back straightened as he watched the man wind a protective arm around Grace's waist. White-hot jealousy seared through Max so quickly he wavered on his feet. The man's skin was the same color as Grace's, offsetting the white of his dress shirt, and the way he stared seemed oddly familiar. The man's dark eyes pinned Max in place before relief and understanding slowly began to settle into Max's bones.

Kai. It had to be her brother.

"Everything's fine," Grace said softly.

"And you are?" Kai uttered, fist clenching on Grace's side.

"I'm Max," Max replied, standing tall, not even remotely in-timidated. "And I'm here to speak to Grace."

"Doesn't seem like she wants to talk to you—"

"Kai, please." She sighed, turning toward her brother.

Max clenched his teeth and looked down at Grace, ignoring her brother's dagger-sharp stare as Grace began to shoo Kai away.

"It's all right," she told her brother. "Really."

Kai huffed. "You're sure?"

"I'm sure."

Kai shot Max another heated look, standing firm at his sister's side, before he made his way back across the gallery.

"I'm sorry," Grace explained when it was just her and Max once more. "He's protective."

"It's okay," Max offered. "I'm glad he is. I just need five minutes. I have to ask—"

"Max," she interrupted, fisting her hands at her stomach. "I know you have things to say, but I'm not ready to . . ." She closed her eyes slowly.

Watching her face crumple as she tried so hard to keep her emotions in check broke Max in two.

What the hell had he been thinking?

He glanced around. His being there was an absolute mistake. He knew with certainty that he was no good for her. He was only human after all and, if they were together he would no doubt fuck up and hurt her again, and no one, least of all Grace, deserved that.

Taking a deep breath that hurt like hell, he risked taking a step closer.

She looked up at him, beautiful and scared.

"I'm sorry," he repeated quietly, memorizing Grace's face. "Truly I am." He ran a hand through his hair. "I just needed to tell you that." He looked around the gallery toward her photographs. "These are really something, Grace."

He reached for her hand, ecstatic that she didn't pull away, and kissed her knuckles gently. "You're amazing. Congratulations."

And with that, Max smiled sadly at her one last time, released her hand, turned, and walked away.

31

Riley dropped Max off at the body shop.

Feeling utterly mauled, Max knew that the smell of gas and oil would keep his mind off the regret gripping him. The ride in the Jeep was silent, yet Max felt Riley's troubled glances on him every couple of seconds.

"You sure you don't want me to take you home, or even to Carter's?" Riley asked, concerned. "Shit, man, you can come back to mine if you want."

Max smiled small and shook his head. "I'm okay," he said, softly unclipping his seat belt. "I just need to be here for a while."

"If you're sure. You call if you need anything," Riley uttered. "I can call Tate—"

"No, I'm fine." He sighed. "I'm not gonna do anything stupid. I know she deserves better than me." He clasped a hand to his friend's shoulder. "I appreciate what you did, though, man."

Riley nodded sharply.

Max climbed out of the Jeep, pulled his keys from his pocket, and unlocked the body shop, then slipped quietly inside. The familiar smells and the cool air immediately calmed a part of Max that yearned for a time when shit was easier; when he was younger, cleaner, and his father was the only thing he had to worry about. He flicked on lights as he went, moving around the three cars the guys had been working on, and made his way to the office. He pushed the leather seat back from the desk and dropped into it, leaning his head back to stare at the ceiling. He closed his eyes against the hurt he'd seen on Grace's face, and breathed.

He meant what he'd said to Riley: Grace deserved better than him. He'd acted like a complete asshole; he'd wounded her, himself, and now he'd lost her. Max wasn't entirely prepared for the sensation of loss that folded through him, but he embraced it all the same. Feeling something was better than feeling nothing at all and, like Tate always said, it reminded Max that he was alive. And, despite all that had happened, including tonight, Max *did* want to be alive.

It was with that last thought that, emotionally exhausted, Max slowly drifted off to sleep.

•   •   •

Max awoke with a start. He groaned when his neck protested at the quick movement, stiff and sore. He rubbed at it and yawned, slightly disoriented, chancing a glance at the clock on the office wall. It was after 1 a.m.

"Shit."

He pulled at his tie, loosening it and pulling it from around his neck, before he undid the top two buttons of his shirt and rolled up the sleeves to his elbows. It was then that he heard a knock. Was that what had woken him?

Cocking his head to listen, the knock came again, this time harder and for longer. Standing on sleepy legs, Max trailed a hand through his hair and approached the door cautiously. Who the hell would be knocking on a body shop door at this time of night? He paused by the side of a large wrench, seriously considering whether or not to pick it up on the off chance that trouble stood on the other side of the door. He grabbed it and leaned it against the side of the wall within easy reach should shit go down. He unlocked the dead bolt, pulled back the second lock, and opened the door a crack.

"Grace."

She stood on the sidewalk, still in her yellow dress. Max opened the door wider. "What are you doing here?"

Grace shook her head. "I don't know."

"Come in." Max stood back as she glanced over her shoulder toward a taxicab that Max belatedly realized was waiting for her. She held up her hand, fingers wide apart, indicating five minutes, and moved past Max into the body shop.

He closed the door behind her. If five minutes was all he had with her, Max knew he couldn't waste a second. "Can I get you anything?"

"No," she answered quickly. "My cab won't wait."

Max dipped his chin in understanding, his head still sleep addled. "Wait. How are you here?" he asked in confusion. "How did you know where I was?"

"Your friend came back to the gallery. He told me where you would be if I changed my mind about speaking to you."

Riley. Well that shit was unexpected. "That's why you're here, you want to talk?" Max hedged.

Grace licked her lips and took a deep breath. "I wanted to know why you came tonight."

Max took a moment to look her over, so spectacular in her dress. "I wanted . . . to see your work. To see you."

"Why?"

Max clenched his teeth, nerves slithering through his veins. "Because I . . . It's been a while since I've seen you, since we've talked, and I wanted to ask you—"

"No," she spat, halting Max's words in their tracks. "You don't understand. You see, I'm fine. Tonight I *was* fine. I *thought* I was fine. And then . . . I saw *you*."

Though he shouldn't have been surprised, hurt sliced through him all the same. "I didn't mean to mess everything up, Grace. I just wanted to make sure you were all right," he stated quietly.

"After I left . . . after what I said." Max pushed his hands into his pockets and kicked gently at an invisible mark on the shop floor. "I just . . ."

"What? What do you want?" she asked, voice soft and expectant.

Max couldn't meet her eyes. "I want . . . I don't want labels. I just want you to be happy, Grace."

"It didn't feel like it the day you left. It felt like I'd been ripped in half." Despite the vehemence in her words, she crossed her arms, clutching her elbows as if holding herself together. "I was ready to let you go—to try and . . . breathe without you."

Her words stole Max's own breath. "I know my apologizing, begging, groveling doesn't take back what I said or how I behaved, but you have to know that none of what I said was true. I didn't mean any of it."

"Then why say it at all?"

Max exhaled heavily and lifted his shoulders. "Because . . . when I arrived in West Virginia, I had this perfect plan. I was quite happy living my life, waking up every fucking day, fighting my demons, my addiction, working with my uncle, moving on as best as I could." He stared at her, so pure and lovely. "And then you . . . you just walked in like a damn hurricane and changed everything."

She looked down toward his feet guiltily. "I didn't mean to. I didn't ever want to—"

"No," he interrupted loudly. "You don't understand, you changed it for the good." He pulled his hands from his pockets and stepped toward her. "I just didn't know what the hell to do. I promised myself that I wouldn't feel anything for anyone ever again and then all of a sudden I was feeling fucking everything at once and I didn't know which way was up. I still don't." Her green eyes lifted to his, tentative and hopeful. "You're like no one I've ever known," he added softly. "You see the good in everything, and everyone, even me."

"But you ran, Max. After everything we'd shared, everything I'd told you, done with you." She shook her head. "I trusted you and you said those awful things when I asked you how you felt."

Max exhaled.

"I know you needed closure, Max. And I hope you got it."

"I did."

She smiled small. "I'm glad. But you were so ready to push me away to get it."

Max groaned in frustration. "I needed space from you to clear my head of what we'd done and how I felt, and coming back here was what I knew. It was the only familiar thing I had among shit that was totally *un*familiar." He gripped his hair before dropping his arms to his sides, defeated. His pulse thundered. "Grace, I—I've never felt what I did that night with you. With anyone."

He chanced a glance at her but her face was unreadable. "But you still hurt me," she whispered.

Max's throat suddenly grew tight as he nodded despondently. He took a stumbling step to the right and rested himself against the side of the cherry-red Mustang. He had no idea where he and Grace went from here. What the hell else was he supposed to say? He had no idea how to fix the damage he'd caused or if she'd even want him to.

"This your father's shop?"

Her question brought his head up, surprised. "Yeah."

"Nice artwork," she said, gesturing to the graffiti that littered the walls. Max had started it last week in an attempt to spruce the place up.

"Thanks," he said. "I thought I'd put my newfound love of painting to good use. It's therapeutic, or so Doc keeps telling me."

Her smile grew a little. She appeared to gather herself before she spoke again. "I promised myself I wouldn't ask you this, because I have absolutely no right to, but, seeing you now, I have to know." She closed her eyes and said, "Did you sleep with her?"

Max's response was immediate and clear. "No."

She reopened her eyes, searching his face for a lie. "Did anything happen?"

Max's gaze drifted to the door, hoping to all hell that she wouldn't leave when he told her the truth. "What happened, Max?"

"When I was leaving," he began, "she asked— We hugged and she kissed me."

"And you kissed her back."

It wasn't a question. "Yes."

She exhaled slowly. "I guess I already knew. She's your first love. I could never compete with that."

"Nobody's asking you to," Max urged. "*I'm* not asking you to."

"No," she murmured. "It just feels that way."

Max stepped closer again, causing Grace to lift her chin to look at him.

"I swear," he insisted. "It was over as quickly as it began and it made me realize that, yes, she was the woman I'd fallen in love with all those years ago, but her lips weren't the ones I wanted. There was nothing there, only memories of a time we'd never get back, and I realized that the man who'd loved her no longer existed."

He lifted a hand and let his finger whisper across her wrist, seeing goose bumps appear instantly. "We're different people, she and I. We want different things. I know now. I know that I need to move forward. I need to look to the future instead of over my fuckin' shoulder waiting for shit to happen; shit that's in the past for a reason."

Resolute, he grabbed her hand, squeezing it tightly as though it would help him keep talking and make her believe what he was saying was true. "I know I hurt you and I'll always be sorry for that. I'll always be an addict but I can't change that, either. All I can do is promise I'll fight it every day. For us. For you."

"Max, I—"

"Do you know what happened when I saw you tonight?" he continued. "After so long . . . You were— Jesus, Gracie, you filled the fucking room. I couldn't see anything but you. I don't crave anything but you." She stared at him. "You told me that all you wanted to do was love me. Am I too late?"

Grace pulled her hand away gently.

"I don't know," she replied, her words firm. "This is a lot to take in, Max. I had no idea. I never thought that you . . ." She shook her head. "I can't be your substitute and I won't be second best."

Max frowned, hating that she'd ever thought that. "You were never second best."

She rubbed the tips of her fingers across her forehead and moved toward the door. She turned back to him. "I can't be a crutch. You have to keep fighting for *you*, Max. No one else."

"I do," he countered. "I will. You just make fighting it that much easier." Her expression softened. "Tell me what you want."

She opened her mouth a couple of times, but no words came. "I don't know."

Max nodded slowly.

"Time," she offered. "I want time to think."

He'd have given her anything she'd asked. "Of course."

She pulled the door open before looking back. "In the gallery and just now, you said you had a question you wanted to ask me. What was it?"

Max smiled small. "It'll keep."

32

It was a week before Max heard from Grace again, a short text asking how he was.

It was ridiculous, really, how seeing her name light up his cell phone screen caused his belly to flutter. He responded in kind, keeping it brief but hopeful, thrilled that they were communicating at all. Max sure as shit hadn't known whether that was even a possibility after the night she'd left him at the body shop.

They texted back and forth for days, until the days turned into another week. It was always casual conversation about how they were spending their time—she was back in Preston County—details about another art show she'd been commissioned for in Philly, following her amazing success in New York, and Max's meetings. Even though he was anxious to ask whether she'd thought any more about what she wanted, he refrained from pushing. Max knew what she was doing. She was learning to trust him again, slowly and surely, opening up and giving him the second chance he so desperately wanted.

And he *was* desperate for it. The more he thought about spending time with her, the more he wanted it. Carter had been right: they didn't need labels. Max just wanted to be with Grace in any capacity she'd allow. In spite of his impatience, Max stayed in New York, resisting the urge to go back to West Virginia, however regretfully, complying with her request for time. It was the least he could do.

Max spent his days doing what he'd always done since he'd left Preston County: running, working, going to his meetings, staying clean, staying sober, fighting the good fight, all the while looking forward to his daily texts from Grace.

It was on a hot evening two weeks after he'd last seen her that Grace called. The conversation wasn't as awkward as Max anticipated. He found himself smiling at the sound of her voice and the excitement she oozed as she told him about her new photographs and filled him in on Uncle Vince and the family, even though she knew Max spoke to them regularly. At first she called twice a week for ten minutes. Then she called three times, until within a week they were speaking for an hour every day. The routine was as easy as it had been when they'd started running together. They fit, not just physically, but emotionally, too.

It was during one of their conversations that Grace brought up the delicate situation of her brother, Kai. Max was under no illusions. He knew that Kai, quite rightly, had taken serious issue with Max's behavior, and as a result he was expressing concern about Grace having any kind of relationship with Max, over the phone or otherwise.

Max was sitting on his sofa, cell phone to his ear, his bare feet kicked up on the coffee table. "Can I do anything to help?" he asked. "I could, I don't know, maybe talk to him."

Grace had laughed nervously. "I'm not sure that's a good idea, but I appreciate the offer. He'll come around. If he knows I'm happy and safe, he'll get over it."

"You're safe with me."

"I know."

Max had swallowed, sensing they were teetering over the line Grace had drawn between the two of them weeks ago. "Do I make you happy?"

She'd paused before saying, "Yes."

Max and Riley threw themselves into organizing Carter's bachelor party, which ended up being a riotous two-day affair in Vegas. Max was more than a little warmed by the fact that Carter, Riley, and of course Tate, whom Max had invited, refrained from drinking in his company. By the second night, however, after a day by the pool, Max forced a tequila into Carter's hand, teasing him mercilessly about how he deserved it for agreeing to subject himself to a life of servitude. There'd been a manly hug and backslap and Carter had knocked that shit back like he'd been desperate for it.

It was followed by five more.

As Carter had requested, there were no strippers, much to Riley's upset. Instead, the ten members of the party enjoyed good food, good wine, scorching-hot weather, and lots and lots of gambling. Max couldn't deny that he'd enjoyed himself, even if it had been hard being in a club not drinking, but his friends were never too far away, encouraging and helping him through it. Max understood that this was how his life would always be, for better or for worse, and as he watched Riley grinding up against a bunch of girls while the others laughed and egged him on, Max realized he was okay with that.

He didn't mind being the designated driver, and he didn't mind helping Carter pull up Kat's cell phone number so that he could call her and tell her how much he was missing her. For one fleeting moment, as Carter rambled and slurred down the phone, and Kat's laughter echoed from the earpiece, Max wondered how Grace would feel if he called to tell her the same.

Three days after they all returned safely to New York, resolute and with a fuck-it-who-cares attitude, Max called Grace and asked her outright, "When can I see you?"

The line was silent for a beat before she replied. "You want to see me?"

Max scoffed and dropped down onto the sofa. "Grace," he sighed. "I *need* to see you." He played with a loose thread hanging from the bottom of his T-shirt. "It's been weeks and I know I said I'd give you time but . . ."

"But what?"

Max cupped a hand to his forehead. "I miss you."

Her breath caught. "I miss you, too."

"Then come," Max insisted, sitting forward. "Come to New York. Or I can come to you, whatever you want."

"How, I'm working? It's Thursday night. Isn't it Carter's wedding this weekend?"

Max smacked a palm against the chair arm. "Fuck." How could he forget that? Some best friend he was. They had a rehearsal dinner tomorrow and then the wedding was Saturday. He still had to run through his best man's speech.

Grace laughed softly. "It's okay."

"Sunday?"

"I can't. I'm in DC with Kai."

Max exhaled heavily and slumped back in his seat. "Next week then."

Grace hummed. "Next week it is."

* * * *

Max could count on his fingers the amount of times he'd seen Carter lose his shit. Despite his reputation, Max's best friend was fairly chill about most things. His wedding day, however, was not one of them. Max couldn't remember seeing Carter so flustered and, honestly, it was funny as fuck.

"Stop laughing and help me, assholes!" Carter exclaimed from his place by a full-length mirror where he'd been battling with his peach-colored tie for at least fifteen minutes. "I'm useless at these fuckin' things."

Max snorted from his spot in the doorway next to Riley and approached, swatting Carter's hands away and tying the tie from behind, his arms reaching over Carter's shoulders. He smiled widely at his friend in the mirror.

"Fuck off," Carter grumbled, rolling his eyes. "I know you love seeing me like this."

"You bet your ass," Max commented. He adjusted the perfect knot of the tie at Carter's throat and patted his friend's belly twice. "Done." Carter exhaled and nodded as Max stepped back.

"Have another drink," Max offered, reaching for a half-filled champagne flute and passing it to him. There were hundreds of them dotted around the beach house, left by the various people milling about. Max wasn't sure he'd ever seen so many busy people.

Carter knocked the drink back and sighed. He glanced at the large watch on his wrist and swallowed audibly. It was showtime in fifteen minutes. Max chuckled and handed him his gray suit jacket. "Dude, relax, you'd think you were due in court."

"No," Carter answered, with a finger pointed in Max's face. "There's no way I'd be this nervous if that was the case."

Both Riley and Max laughed. Max glanced back at Riley, who, understanding the need for the two best friends to have a moment, nodded and snuck out of the room, closing the door behind him.

"What are you so nervous about, man?" Max asked, looking back at Carter, who placed his empty glass down on a nearby shelf and shrugged into his jacket. "Isn't this what you want?"

"Yes!" Carter blurted. "Yes, of course, I can't wait to see her, to marry her, but . . ." He glanced at the window, out toward the beach where rows of chairs were filling with people and a white archway decorated in white and peach-colored flowers stood in front of a very official-looking man, all waiting for the wedding to begin.

"You're just scared about fucking up?"

Carter nodded and whispered, "Shitless."

Max smiled and stepped closer to his best friend. "You've got this, brother. Okay? She loves you. Fuck knows why"—they both chuckled—"but she does." He squeezed Carter's shoulder. "So go down there and show everyone why she chose you."

Carter's eyes glistened in a way that made Max shift on his feet. "I'm proud of you, Max," he said softly. "So fucking proud."

Max had no time to reply before Carter pulled him into a tight hug. There were no backslaps, no manly declarations, just two men with twenty years of friendship between them, silently appreciating how far they'd both come.

Carter never wavered after that.

Max stood proudly at his side, where he'd always been and would always be, as Carter married Kat, who was stunning in her ivory dress. The vows they both spoke were moving and said with such fervency that, a few times, Max's chest echoed with a pang of longing for Grace. Nevertheless, Max was the first to stand, clap, and cheer when Kat and Carter had their first kiss as husband and wife.

Outside the beach house, on the sand, a dance floor and bar area had been constructed, surrounded by white tables where the wedding party ate their meal and toasted the bride and groom. The lapping ocean was the only sound track to Max's best man's speech, before the DJ invited the newlyweds onto the floor for their first dance. Watching the happy couple dance to Otis Redding, Max recalled dancing with Grace in the godforsaken bar Ruby had taken them to that July weekend and smiled quietly to himself at the memory. She'd looked so damned beautiful that night.

Riley thumped down next to Max as the dance floor started to fill up. "Sweet speech. You did good, man," he uttered, his eyes on a young brunette dancing not ten feet away.

Max grinned. "Thanks, dude."

Riley looked over at him and winked. "So, you and running girl—you ready for all this?" He gestured toward where Kat and Carter swayed slowly amid the other, more exuberant dancers on the floor; the newlyweds were staring at one another as though the entire world had stopped around them.

Max shook his head. "Not a wedding."

He watched as Carter's head fell back, laughing loudly at something Kat had said. Max's chest tightened with undeniable joy for his friend, which was swiftly followed by a Grace-shaped ache. "But being happy? Yeah, I'm more than ready for that."

"Amen, brother," Riley murmured, turning from where Brunette was making heart eyes at him, and rested his elbows on the tabletop.

Max mirrored him. "You okay?"

Riley nodded, loosening his tie and popping open the top button of his shirt. "Yeah. It's just . . . sometimes I wonder where I would be if I'd made a different decision, you know?"

Although Max wasn't aware of the decision Riley spoke of, he knew all too well what that feeling of regret was like, and he hated the thought of his friend feeling anything even remotely close to it. Riley's hazel eyes were troubled.

"You wanna talk about it?"

Riley smiled, but it was fleeting. "Nah, man." He lifted his drink and tapped it against Max's glass of Dr Pepper. "Today's for celebrating, not commiserating." He knocked back the champagne and stood with his arms out wide. "Dancing time!"

Max snorted as he watched Riley shuffle and bop onto the dance floor toward Brunette, shrugging out of his suit jacket as he did. It always amazed Max how resilient Riley seemed to be. Tate was right, he was just like a bouncy ball, but still Max worried.

With his soda in hand, Max wandered around the dance floor, smiling and speaking to friends and members of Kat's family. Her mother was a little prickly, as Carter had warned him she might be, but her stepfather seemed cool. Her grandmother, Nana Boo, though, was fucking epic and danced with Max for two full songs before she went off in search of a glass of sherry. It eased a small part of Max knowing that Carter had a new family around him, people who seemed to genuinely care and want good things for him and Kat.

He looked out at the ocean, as blue as the sky it met on the horizon, and closed his eyes knowing that Grace would have loved it. He would have loved dancing here with her, in the moonlight, kissing her under the stars.

"Max?" Startled, he turned to see Kat, cheeks flushed, her green eyes bright and happy. "You okay?"

He smiled, shaking off the whispers of melancholy his thoughts of Grace brought. "Yeah. I'm good. How're you?" He nodded toward where Carter was dancing with Nana Boo, her small bare feet balanced on his large shiny dress shoes. "Feel weird yet?"

Kat laughed. "No. It feels perfect."

"Good."

"You sure you're still okay staying here tonight after we leave?"

He sipped his drink. "Absolutely."

"Great." She smirked, glancing at him out of the corner of her eye. "You know, I was thinking, maybe you could ask Grace to stay here with you."

Max frowned, having thought about the exact same thing and how awesome it would have been. "She's in Preston County," he muttered.

"Really?" Kat looked back at him and tilted her head toward the house.

Max's gaze snapped over to the beach house, where, standing by the French windows, in the same red dress she'd worn at the lake, was Grace. His chest did an honest-to-God somersault when she smiled nervously, causing him to stare, knowing she was damn near the most perfect thing he'd ever seen.

Max wasn't sure how he got to her, wasn't sure whether he walked or floated across the dance floor, and only realized he was moving when he was a couple of feet away from her. He stopped, taking her in, her black hair loose around her face and down her back and shoulders, fluttering in the gentle breeze. Her beautiful dark skin, exquisite against the vibrant color of her dress, and her long legs, perfect feet, and toes that were painted to match.

He licked his lips. "What—how—what are . . . ?"

She laughed. "Does it matter?"

He shook his head, stuck for words. "No. It doesn't matter one bit. You're here. I thought . . ."

"I thought so, too, but . . . I missed you too much." She gestured toward his gray suit with a lift of her hand. "You look beautiful."

Max grimaced. "That was going to be my line."

Smirking, Grace shrugged. "Well, it's my line now." She laughed again when Max stayed silent, unable to do anything but just look at her. "What?"

"Just you," he answered, taking a step closer. "Fillin' the fuckin' room."

"I'm in the doorway," she teased. "I'm practically outside."

"Doesn't matter where you are," he assured her. "You're all I see."

Grace's face seemed to soften and relax with his words. "Max." She stepped forward, closing the remaining distance between them, the scent of cocoa butter wafting over him. "Before we say or do anything else, we have to talk."

Max nodded, his pulse spiking with anticipation, not knowing whether to laugh or cry.

"You asked me to tell you what I want," she continued. "And I can tell you now."

"Okay." Max braced himself.

Grace licked her top lip, scraping it gently with her teeth, as her shoulders rose. "I want you to tell me that this is real," she said carefully. "I want you to tell me you want this; that you want me; not that you need me, because you don't need me any more than you need to drink or get high. I want you to promise me that you're not going to run away again, that you'll talk, be honest with me, that we'll both always fight our demons for ourselves, not each other. And, if you can, if you can do all of that, I'll swear to you, I'll do the same."

Max swallowed as her request wrapped tightly around his heart, trapping his reply in his throat. He breathed, clenched his teeth in an effort to gather himself, and said, "I won't run again. Ever. And I do want you. I do, Grace. This is *real*, I promise. I lo— I . . ."

Grace squeezed his hand, halting his struggle with words he hadn't uttered to anyone for a hell of a long time. "No labels," she murmured, smiling.

His shoulders dropped in relief. It wasn't that Max didn't *want* to say the words. Jesus, he wanted to tell her; he just didn't know if he could. They'd frightened him beyond reason for so long that, despite feeling what they stood for in every fiber of his body, voicing them to Grace would take time.

"Don't worry," Grace added, as if reading his mind. "It'll come. Don't be afraid."

"I'm terrified," Max admitted, repeating his words from the last time they'd made love.

"I know. Me, too. But we'll find our way." She entwined their fingers. "Together."

He dropped his forehead gently to hers, closing his eyes as the weight of what they were choosing pressed on him deliciously, like a winter blanket.

"Tell me something," she said quietly.

"Anything."

"What was your question? The night at the gallery, what did you want to ask me?"

Max lifted his head. He raised a hand and cupped the side of Grace's face, smiling when she leaned into it. His thumb wandered lazily over the apple of her cheek, across her soft skin.

"You said you understood that Lizzie was my first love," he murmured. "And you were right, she was."

Grace nodded, her expression solemn. "I know."

Max stilled. "And my question for you was: Would you be my last?"

Grace gasped a breath that quickly shuddered out of her. Her mouth lifted into the most gorgeous of smiles, as she shivered under Max's fingertips. She closed her eyes, tears sitting in the corners of them. "On one condition," she said, looking up at him.

Max smirked but schooled his features quickly, playing along. "Okay, Gracie. What's the condition?"

"That you kiss me," she answered without hesitation.

"Right now?"

"Right now."

Max glanced at her glorious mouth, slightly open, lips wet, and cocked an eyebrow, pretending to consider it. She narrowed her eyes playfully but, before she could say anything, Max cupped the other side of her face, leaned down, and kissed her. She hummed into him, grasping his arms, causing Max to lose himself in her taste and her touch all over again.

He was vaguely aware of cheering and whoops that sounded suspiciously like Riley, Tate, and Carter, but he couldn't have cared less.

All he cared about was the woman wrapped in his arms, whispering her love for him, and the overwhelming sensation of hope that began to bloom among all the parts of him that belonged to his Grace.

Wes Carter: Dangerous, brooding and behind bars, Carter's emotional scars are as permanent as the ink on his skin.

Kat Lane: Vibrant and gutsy, Kat chooses to become a prison tutor in tribute to her father whose murder haunts her.

As teacher and student, any relationship is against every rule. But although their love is forbidden, it won't be denied . . .

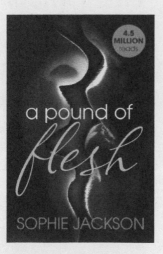

Available now from

headline
ETERNAL

Theirs was a love that broke every rule. The searing attraction between Wes Carter and Kat Lane was instant and impossible to deny.

But as they face real life together and share the news of their engagement with those closest to them, Kat and Carter realise that they will still have to fight for their love if it is to survive forever and . . . always.

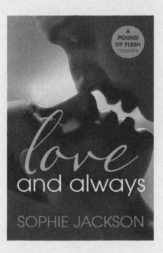

Available now as an e-novella from

headline
ETERNAL

headline
ETERNAL

FIND YOUR HEART'S DESIRE...

VISIT OUR WEBSITE: www.headlineeternal.com
FIND US ON FACEBOOK: facebook.com/eternalromance
FOLLOW US ON TWITTER: @eternal_books
EMAIL US: eternalromance@headline.co.uk